Recent Progress in Endoscopic Surgery

Recent Progress in Endoscopic Surgery

Edited by **Steven Notley**

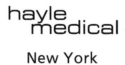

New York

Published by Hayle Medical,
30 West, 37th Street, Suite 612,
New York, NY 10018, USA
www.haylemedical.com

Recent Progress in Endoscopic Surgery
Edited by Steven Notley

© 2015 Hayle Medical

International Standard Book Number: 978-1-63241-335-2 (Hardback)

Printed in the United States of America.

Contents

Preface

I am honored to present to you this unique book which encompasses the most up-to-date data in the field. I was extremely pleased to get this opportunity of editing the work of experts from across the globe. I have also written papers in this field and researched the various aspects revolving around the progress of the discipline. I have tried to unify my knowledge along with that of stalwarts from every corner of the world, to produce a text which not only benefits the readers but also facilitates the growth of the field.

This book unifies the current concepts and advanced researches in the field of endoscopic surgery. Surgeons from varied domains have become extremely interested in endoscopy, with its low complication rates, high analytic yields and the opportunity to carry out a large diversity of therapeutic techniques. In the past few decades, the variety of surgical endoscopic methods has developed with many new techniques for both analysis and management, and these developments are presented in this book. This book discusses various concepts related to endoscopic surgery. It also elucidates various branches of endoscopic surgery such as digestive, urogynecological and pediatric endoscopy. Contributing to the expansion of endoscopic surgery around the world, this is a contemporary, informational, and interesting book which presents the current developments in this field.

Finally, I would like to thank all the contributing authors for their valuable time and contributions. This book would not have been possible without their efforts. I would also like to thank my friends and family for their constant support.

Editor

Part 1

Digestive Endoscopy

Surgical Treatment of Gastroesophageal Reflux Disease

Filippo Tosato[1], Salvatore Marano[1],
Stefano Mattacchione[1], Barbara Luongo[1],
Giulia Paltrinieri[1], Valentina Mingarelli[1]
and Leoluca Vasapollo[2]
[1]Referral Center for the Surgical Treatment
of Gastroesophageal Reflux Diseases,
"Sapienza" University of Rome
[2]Sandro Pertini Hospital, Rome
Italy

1. Introduction

Gastro-esophageal reflux disease (GERD) is "a condition which develops when the reflux of stomach contents causes troublesome symptoms (i.e., at least two heartburn episodes per week) and/or complications" (Vakil et al 2006) and represents one of the fastest growing disease affecting the alimentary tract. Recently studies on the epidemiology of GERD demonstrating that GERD is a highly prevalent disorder with 10-20% of individuals affected in western civilization (Dent et al 2005). When GERD is defined as twice weekly reflux over several months, 10-20% of individuals in Western civilization are affected, which is significantly higher than in Asian population (5%) (Bonatti et al 2008). In a large prospective American cohort study is reported that 25% of investigated individuals experienced nocturnal reflux symptoms (Fass et al 2005). A recent population-based study demonstrated the prevalence of reflux symptoms to be 44% with 24% of individuals experiencing symptoms for two days or more per week. The prevalence of oesophagitis and Barrett's oesophagus was 12% and 1.3% respectively, irrespective of symptoms (Zagari et al 2008).Thirty-three per cent of individuals with oesophagitis and 46% with Barrett's oesophagus were asymptomatic. Severe GERD can lead to potentially avoidable complications including severe oesophagitis with scarring and stricture formation, Barrett's esophagus and adenocarcinoma.When symptoms become frequent and severe enough to require regular medication, there is a significant impact on quality of life (Ware et al 1992).(QOL)

2. Pathophysiology

GERD results from failure of the reflux barrier. This barrier has three components: (1) an intra-abdominal esophagus of adequate length, (2) an extrinsic sphincter, the esophageal hiatus, and (3) an intrinsic sphincter, the lower esophageal sphincter (Bloom et al 2009).

Relaxation of the LES and crura are normal physiological processes occurring during swallowing and also during gas venting. Relaxations not initiated by a swallow are known as transient lower esophageal relaxations (TLESRs). Abnormal TLESRs have a greater crosssectional area at the gastro-oesophageal junction resulting in the reflux of gastric fluid in addition to gas. TLESRs probably account for 90% of reflux episodes. The TLESR reflex is initiated by tension receptors in the stomach and mediated by a vagovagal pathway via the brainstem leading to simultaneous relaxation of the crura, LES and inhibition of peristalsis (Pandolfino et al 2003). These responses are inhibited by gammaaminobutyric acid-B (GABA-B) receptor agonists, and thus may constitute a future therapeutic target. Hiatus hernias appear to increase the magnitude of reflux during TLESRs. Transient lower oesophageal relaxations appear to be less significant in more severe reflux esophagitis. A hypotensive LES, which allows high pressure gradients across the diaphragm, is probably responsible for more severe esophagitis (Barham et al 1995). Reflux occurs more frequently when the pressure in the LES is <10 mm Hg, and free reflux only occursif the LES pressure is <4 mm Hg (Kahrilas et al 1986; Dodds et al 1982). Factors which relax the LES, such as caffeine, fat, smoking, drugs (calcium channel antagonists and nitrates) and gastric distention, will increase the likelihood of reflux. The association of increased body mass index and GERD remains unclear (Hampel et al 2005; Pandolfino et al 2006). A recent study failed to demonstrate an increased risk of reflux symptoms or esophagitis in obese individuals. Acid in the distal oesophagus has been shown to be neutralised by saliva. Therefore any processes reducing saliva production results in a delay in acid neutralisation. Nocturnal reflux episodes are prolonged due to depressed salivation. Acid is cleared by oesophageal peristalsis. Therefore impaired distal esophageal peristalsis results in prolonged acid exposure to acid reflux episodes. This is apparent in both hiatus hernias and ulcerative oesophagitis where there is peristaltic dysfunction (Kahrilas et al 2006, Johnson et al 1980).

3. Simptomatology

Typical GERD symptoms—heartburn and regurgitation—reflect dysfunction of the reflux barrier.
Dysphagia is a third, less specific, GERD symptom. It may be caused by GERD itself or stricture complicating GERD. GERD-related dysphagia must be differentiated from functional and mechanical dysphagia resulting from multiple other diseases that cause symptomatic esophageal obstruction. Atypical GERD symptoms are cough, asthma, laryngitis, sore throat, chest pain, abdominal pain, and bloating. These symptoms in the absence of typical GERD symptoms point to diseases other than GERD. Careful investigation of alternative causes of atypical symptoms is necessary. Sophisticated testing, including impedance/pH monitoring, must be performed if GERD is believed to be the cause of atypical symptoms and surgery is being considered (Bajbouj et al 2007; Fornari et al 2007). Comparing international literature with our case studies we can confirm that number of patients with atypical symptoms referring to our Referral Center for the Surgical Treatment of Gastroesophageal Reflux Diseases is growing. In fact 644 patients (30.7%), who underwent to endoscopic exams, showed typical and atypical symptoms (heartburn, pyrosis, regurgitation, asthma, laryngospasm, pulmonary fibrosis), and 96 patients (4.6%) had only atypical symptoms.

Reflux esophagitis is defined as reflux causing inflammation or ulceration of the esophagus. Attempts have been made to classify the extent of damage, of which the Los Angeles classification is now the most commonly used:

Grade	Extent of esophageal inflammation
A	Mucosal breaks<5mm not extending between folds
B	Mucosal breaks>5mm not extending between folds
C	Mucosal breaks extending between folds
D	Mucosal breaks extending between > 2 folds involving > 75% of the circumference

4. Diagnosis

The signs and symptoms are insufficient to establish a conclusive diagnosis of GERD, regardless of their frequency and intensity, resulting in a diagnostic certainty of around 40%. Endoscopy is not usually performed in young adults patients with typical history of GERD since it does not alter the clinical evolution when compared to the empiric treatment.

In patients with non-erosive GERD, the use of the symptom score (moderate or severe) allows a diagnostic certainty of up to 40% of the cases. In these cases, the upper digestive endoscopy (UDE) does not alter the clinical evolution, when compared to the empiric treatment. It is interesting to remember that, in cases of erosive GERD with typical symptoms, however, the UDE improves the diagnostic accuracy and also establishes a differential diagnosis with other diseases, such as cancer. The 24-hour pH-metry is the most important resource for a definite diagnosis of acid reflux, which constitutes most of reflux episodes, establishing or ruling out the diagnosis with a 90% and 95% certainty, respectively. Actually the acid component of the gastric refluxate is responsible for most of the symptoms and pathology associated with GERD, however, other components, such as bile, may also contribute (known as nonacidreflux). Quantification of reflux can be achieved either by measuring acid exposure to the distal esophagus (pH studies) or movement of liquid in the distal esophagus (impedance studies). Combined impedance and pH measurement characterizes all acid and non-acid reflux episodes.

Nearly 70% of patients with heartburn do not have evidence of erosive changes on endoscopy. Of these, a proportion have increased acid reflux on 24-hour pH monitoring and are classified as having non-erosive reflux disease (NERD) (Jones et al 1995).

In patients with atypical manifestations, the conventional esophageal pH-metry contributes little to the diagnosis of GERD. The current available evidence does not support the routine use of proximal pH monitoring. In patients with atypical manifestations, the impedance-pH-metry substantially contributes to the diagnosis of GERD. In patients undergoing prolonged treatment with PPI, the histological esophageal alterations can remain practically unaltered, regardless of the occurrence or not of symptoms and signs. On the other hand, the histological alterations accompany the degree of severity of the esophagitis. Therefore, the evaluation of the histological signs increases the diagnostic probability of GERD. The observation of the dimensions of the distal esophagus intercellular space increases the probability of diagnostic certainty and also allows the analysis of the therapeutic response. Esophageal biopsies in patients with suspected GERD for the analysis of basal cell proliferation allow, in absence of the latter, ruling out the diagnosis or active disease. The isolated presence of the basal layer proliferation, however, has little diagnostic value. Although the basal cell thickness allows the analysis of the therapeutic response, it is not correlated with the clinical response. The presence of reflux symptoms in asthmatic patients results in a small increase in the probability of diagnostic certainty. In asthmatic patients with reflux symptoms, the normal pH-metry can predict the absence of therapeutic response with PPI. A significant number of patients with asthma (57%) also present gastroesophageal reflux.GERD may also produce esophageal injury. Esophagogastroduodenoscopy (EGD) with biopsy has replaced the upright air-contrast phase of the barium esophagram for mucosa evaluation. EGD and biopsy both diagnose and assess esophageal injury by visual and histopathologic mucosal examination. Visual assessment of esophageal injury is graded using the Los Angeles classification. Histopathologic findings, although nonspecific, are confirmatory in the clinical setting of GERD. The finding of specialized columnar epithelium (Barrett esophagus) in the tubular esophagus is secondary to GERD. In the absence of dysplasia, surveillance esophagoscopy and biopsy are required in patients who have Barrett esophagus, regardless of therapy (medical or surgical).

If dysphagia is the predominant symptom and the diagnosis is in question, the examination should start as a timed barium esophagram.

Esophageal manometry excludes unsuspected motility disorders or motility disorders masquerading as GERD, confirms adequate esophageal peristalsis for GERD surgery, and quantifies preoperative resting pressure and relaxation of the lower esophageal sphincter for later comparison. It must be considered in all surgical patients when clinically or ph-metrically a motility disorder is suspected.

5. Management

The aim of GERD treatment is to effectively control symptoms and prevent GERD-associated complications. As with many conditions, adopting a stepped approach to treatment helps tailor disease severity to treatment regimen.

5.1 Lifestyle changes
Simple manoeuvres may have a marked effect on symptoms. These are outlined below:
- dietary changes. Some substances influence oesophageal physiology favouring increased acid   reflux. These include fat, caffeine and alcohol
- avoiding late meals. Acid reflux episodes are prolonged when asleep as a result of both gravity, and also reduced peristalsis and acid clearance. Nocturnal reflux can therefore be minimised by consuming small meals long before sleep
- although the association of obesity and GERD is unclear, there does appear to be an association with esophageal adenocarcinoma and many other well-known diseases.11 On this basis weight loss is suggested as part of GERD management.

5.2 Antacids/alginate combinations
Antacids consist of calcium carbonate, magnesium and aluminum salts in various compounds or combinations. The effect of antacids is due to partial neutralization of gastric hydrochloric acid and inhibition of the proteolytic enzyme, pepsin. Alginate mechanism of action is due to the formation of a gel in the presence of gastric acid. Alginate-based reforming formulations usually contain sodium or potassium bicarbonate; in the presence of gastric acid, the bicarbonate is converted to carbon dioxide, which becomes entrapped within the gel precipitate, converting it into a foam which floats on the surface of the gastric

contents, much like a raft on water. Both *in vitro* and *in vivo* studies have demonstrated that alginate-based rafts can entrap carbon dioxide, as well as antacid components contained in some formulations, thus providing a relatively pH neutral barrier. Antacids and alginates have been shown to improve reflux symptoms, however, they do not heal oesophagitis (Stanciu et 1974). They are indicated for very mild symptoms, where step-up treatment is not necessary. There is no role for antacids/alginates in the maintenance of GERD.

Despite the development of potent medications for the treatment of GERD, antacids remain a mainstay of treatment. Antacids neutralize the acid in the stomach so that there is no acid to reflux. The problem with antacids is that their action is brief. They are emptied from the empty stomach quickly, in less than an hour, and the acid then re-accumulates. The best way to take antacids, therefore, is approximately one hour after meals or just before the symptoms of reflux begin after a meal. Since the food from meals slows the emptying from the stomach, an antacid taken after a meal stays in the stomach longer and is effective longer. For the same reason, a second dose of antacids approximately two hours after a meal takes advantage of the continuing post-meal slower emptying of the stomach and replenishes the acid-neutralizing capacity within the stomach.

Antacids may be aluminum, magnesium, or calcium based. Calcium-based antacids (usually calcium carbonate), unlike other antacids, stimulate the release of gastrin from the stomach and duodenum. Gastrin is the hormone that is primarily responsible for the stimulation of acid secretion by the stomach. Therefore, the secretion of acid rebounds after the direct acid-neutralizing effect of the calcium carbonate is exhausted. The rebound is due to the release of gastrin, which results in an overproduction of acid. Theoretically at least, this increased acid is not good for GERD.

Acid rebound, however, has not been shown to be clinically important. That is, treatment with calcium carbonate has not been shown to be less effective or safe than treatment with antacids not containing calcium carbonate. Nevertheless, the phenomenon of acid rebound is theoretically harmful. In practice, therefore, calcium-containing antacids such as Tums and Rolaids are not recommended. The occasional use of these calcium carbonate-containing antacids, however, is not believed to be harmful. The advantages of calcium carbonate-containing antacids are their low cost , the calcium they add to the diet, and their convenience as compared to liquids.

Aluminum-containing antacids have a tendency to cause constipation, while magnesium-containing antacids tend to cause diarrhea. If diarrhea or constipation becomes a problem, it may be necessary to switch antacids or alternately use antacids containing aluminum and magnesium.

5.3 Histamine antagonists
Although antacids can neutralize acid, they do so for only a short period of time. For substantial neutralization of acid throughout the day, antacids would need to be given frequently, at least every hour. The first medication developed for more effective and convenient treatment of acid-related diseases, including GERD, was a histamine antagonist, specifically cimetidine. H2 antagonists are very good for relieving the symptoms of GERD, particularly heartburn. However, they are not very good for healing the inflammation (esophagitis) that may accompany GERD. In fact, they are used primarily for the treatment of heartburn in GERD that is not associated with inflammation or complications, such as erosions or ulcers, strictures, or Barrett's esophagus. Four

different H2 antagonists are available by prescription, including cimetidine, ranitidine, nizatidine, and famotidine. All four are also available over-the-counter (OTC), without the need for a prescription. However, the OTC dosages are lower than those available by prescription. Histamine is an important chemical because it stimulates acid production by the stomach. Released within the wall of the stomach, histamine attaches to receptors (binders) on the stomach's acid-producing cells and stimulates the cells to produce acid. Histamine antagonists work by blocking the receptor for histamine and thereby preventing histamine from stimulating the acid-producing cells. (Histamine antagonists are referred to as H2 antagonists because the specific receptor they block is the histamine type 2 receptor.) Because histamine is particularly important for the stimulation of acid after meals, H2 antagonists are best taken 30 minutes before meals. The reason for this timing is so that the H2 antagonists will be at peak levels in the body after the meal when the stomach is actively producing acid. H2 antagonists also can be taken at bedtime to suppress nighttime production of acid.

5.4 Proton pump inhibitors

The second type of drug developed specifically for acid-related diseases, such as GERD, was a proton pump inhibitor (PPI), specifically, omeprazole. A PPI blocks the secretion of acid into the stomach by the acid-secreting cells. Proton pump inhibitors (PPIs) bind to enzymes in the stomach membrane that produce hydrochloric acid. PPIs reduce levels of stomach acid, and are commonly used to reduce acid reflux symptoms, heal ulcers, and treat gastroesophageal reflux disease (GERD).The advantage of a PPI over an H2 antagonist is that the PPI shuts off acid production more completely and for a longer period of time. Not only is the PPI good for treating the symptom of heartburn, but it also is good for protecting the esophagus from acid so that esophageal inflammation can heal. PPIs are used when H2 antagonists do not relieve symptoms adequately or when complications of GERD such as erosions or ulcers, strictures, or Barrett's esophagus exist. Five different PPIs are approved for the treatment of GERD, including omeprazole, lansoprazole, rabeprazole, pantoprazole, and esomeprazole. A fifth PPI product consists of a combination of omeprazole and sodium bicarbonate. PPIs are best taken an hour before meals. The reason for this timing is that the PPIs work best when the stomach is most actively producing acid, which occurs after meals. If the PPI is taken before the meal, it is at peak levels in the body after the meal when the acid is being made. Esomeprazole 20/40 mg/day, lansoprazole 30 mg/day, omeprazole 20/40 mg/day, pantoprazole 40 mg/day and rabeprazole 20 mg/day are equivalent in the treatment of patients with erosive and non-erosive GERD. The report of the occurrence of neoplasia with the chronic use of PPI is not supported by evidence. The gastric mucosa, however, is altered in these conditions (chronic gastritis, atrophy and polyps of fundic glands). The prevalence of gastric atrophy signs increases along the years, mainly when *H. pylori* is present.

At the primary care level, PPI or a combination of alginate-antacid and acid suppressive therapy can be administered at the discretion of the physician, as combination therapy, which may potentially be more beneficial than acid suppressive therapy alone. Similarly, patients who fail full-dose PPIs, plus/minus adjuvant therapies, may benefit from step-up therapy to twice daily PPIs even if there is no difference in randomized studies regarding the clinical response to the treatment with PPI taken as two daily doses, when compared to a single daily dose.

When the PPI were used in full dose (esomeprazole: 20 mg/day and 40 mg/day; lansoprazole: 15 mg/day and 30 mg/day; omeprazole: 40 mg/day; pantoprazole 20 mg/day and 40 mg/day; rabeprazole: 10 mg/day and 20 mg/day), no statistical difference was observed between 4 and 8 weeks of treatment. Nevertheless, in cases of therapeutic failure, the time of treatment can be extended from 4 to 8 weeks, as although no significant difference was observed between the two periods, the number of satisfactory responses is higher after 8 than after 4 weeks.

5.5 Pro-motility drugs
Pro-motility drugs work by stimulating the muscles of the gastrointestinal tract, including the esophagus, stomach, small intestine, and/or colon. One pro-motility drug, metoclopramide, is approved for GERD. Pro-motility drugs increase the pressure in the lower esophageal sphincter and strengthen the contractions (peristalsis) of the esophagus. Both effects would be expected to reduce reflux of acid. However, these effects on the sphincter and esophagus are small. Therefore, it is believed that the primary effect of metoclopramide may be to speed up emptying of the stomach, which also would be expected to reduce reflux. Pro-motility drugs are most effective when taken 30 minutes before meals and again at bedtime. They are not very effective for treating either the symptoms or complications of GERD. Therefore, the pro-motility agents are reserved either for patients who do not respond to other treatments or are added to enhance other treatments for GERD.

5.6 Foam barriers
Foam barriers provide a unique form of treatment for GERD. Foam barriers are tablets that are composed of an antacid and a foaming agent. As the tablet disintegrates and reaches the stomach, it turns into foam that floats on the top of the liquid contents of the stomach. The foam forms a physical barrier to the reflux of liquid. At the same time, the antacid bound to the foam neutralizes acid that comes in contact with the foam. The tablets are best taken after meals (when the stomach is distended) and when lying down, both times when reflux is more likely to occur. Foam barriers are not often used as the first or only treatment for GERD. Rather, they are added to other drugs for GERD when the other drugs are not adequately effective in relieving symptoms. There is only one foam barrier, which is a combination of aluminum hydroxide gel, magnesium trisilicate, and alginate.

6. Surgery

When the diagnosis of reflux is objectively confirmed, surgical therapy should be considered in individuals who (Rice et al 2008):
1. have failed medical management (inadequate symptom control, severe regurgitation not controlled with acidsuppression, or medication side effects)
OR
2. opt for surgery despite successful medical management (due to quality of life considerations, lifelong need for medication intake, expense of medications, etc.)
OR
3. have complications of GERD (e.g., Barrett's esophagus, peptic stricture) (Spechler et 1996; Lagergren et al 1999)

OR
4. have extra-esophageal manifestations (asthma, hoarseness, cough, chest pain, aspiration) (Rakita et al 2006; Oelshlager et al 2002).

The coexistence of Barrett's esophagus with gastroesophageal reflux symptoms is considered by many a clear indication for antireflux surgery (Oelshlager et al 2002). Surgical intervention for asymptomatic Barrett's esophagus is more controversial, however. While the metaplastic changes of Barrett's have been reported to regress to a greater degree in the post-surgical population compared with medically treated patients, to date there is no demonstrable improvement in esophageal adenocarcinoma rates (Rossi et al 2006; Chang et al 2007).

Today there is increased tendency worldwide to utilize surgery in the earlier stages of the disease (Spechler et al 2001). This change in clinical practice is mainly due to advancements in surgical technique, the increased patient satisfaction by laparoscopy, and the increased awareness of the impairment in quality of life of patients who are not efficiently treated. Moreover, the increasing enthusiasm of patients and surgeons for minimally invasive surgery has led to the wider application of laparoscopy in the management of GERD in many institutes worldwide.

The large success of laparoscopic surgery as an effective treatment of gastroesophageal reflux disease, has established minimal invasive surgery as the gold standard in the surgical treatment of this condition.

The guidelines from American Society for Gastrointestinal and Endoscopic Surgeons (SAGES) claim that surgery in GERD is curative in 85-93% of cases and suggest that the procedure may be appropriate in patients who have failed medical management, decide for surgery despite successful medical management, have complication of GERD, have medical complications attributable to a large hiatal hernia, or have "atypical" symptoms and reflux documented on 24h pH monitoring (SAGES Guidelines 2010).

Antireflux surgery has been shown to be very effective in relieving symptoms in 88-95% of patients, with excellent patients satisfaction, both in short and long term studies (Laffularde et al 2001; McKenzie et al 1996).

There are several trials favoring the clinical outcome of laparoscopic antireflux surgery compared to long-term PPI therapy. A large randomized clinical trial from the UK has shown significantly better physiological control of reflux in patients having undergone laparoscopic Nissen fundoplication than patients under maintenance PPI therapy (Laffularde et al 2001).

A randomized trial with 5-year follow-up, demonstrated that antireflux surgery is more effective than proton pomp inhibitor (PPI) drugs in controlling GERD symptoms (Laffularde et al 2001; Lundell et al 2001).

At 7-years follow-up Lundell et all reported the results of a randomized controlled trial of patients with esophagitis treated with omeprazole or surgery. The two treatments were similar regarding the incidence of recurrent esophagitis (10.3% omeprazole versus 11.8% antireflux surgery). In addition the two therapies appeared to be equivalent in healing esophageal mucosa (Lundell et al 2007).

Another randomized trial, with 10 year follow-up, evaluating the effectiveness of medical therapy (omeprazole) versus antireflux surgery found that patients who underwent surgery had improved symptoms' relief when compared to the medically treated group (Spechler et al 2001).

After 1991 when Dallemagne et al (Dallemagne et al 1991)performed the first laparoscopic Nissen Fundoplication, this technique was preferred to open procedures to result in lower morbidity and mortality, shorter hospital stay, faster recovery and less postoperative pain.

In a review by Catarci et al, laparoscopic fundoplication was as effective as its open counterpart with reduced morbidity, shorter hospital stay, and recovery but without any significant difference in early functional results and outcome (Catarci et al 2004).

Salminen et al in a recent randomized controlled trial, with 11-year follow-up, compared laparoscopic approach and conventional Nissen Fundoplication and concluded that the open and laparoscopic approaches for the Nissen fundoplication have similar long-term subjective symptomatic outcome despite the significantly higher evidence of incisional hernia and defective fundic wraps at endoscopy in the open group (Salminen et al 2007).

In a recent review Peters and colleagues compared 503 laparoscopic anti-reflux surgery and 533 open anti-reflux surgery. In this meta-analysis the authors conclude that laparoscopic anti-reflux surgery enables a faster convalescence and return to productive activity, with a reduced risk of complications and a similar treatment outcome compared with that of the open approach (Peters et al 2009).

The surgical management of GERD has been difficult to study scientifically because of the significant variation in the surgical techniques used.

The LOTUS trial (Attwood et al 2008)was designed to identify a methodology for standardization of the surgical technique and to measure the effectiveness of this standardization. This study has shown that surgeons are able to standardize their work for the purpose of measuring the outcome of an operative procedure within the context of a randomized trial.

Several series have shown the early outcomes of laparoscopic Nissen fundoplication to be excellent, with minimal morbidity and mortality, marked reduction in distal esophageal acid exposure, and symptom control for the overwhelming majority of patients. There have been multiple series with 5-year outcomes following Laparoscopic Nissen Fundoplication (Table 1). Heartburn was controlled in approximately 90% of patients, the revision rate was between 1 and 17%, and 86%-92% of patients that were off antireflux medications.

In the German experience, in 164 hospitals performing laparoscopic antireflux surgery and 2053 operation were reported in 1999. In 65% of the cases the surgical procedures were total fundoplication, in 31% partial fundoplication and in 4% other techniques. In total fundoplication there were 5 different techniques, in partial plication 5 and in the other group 3 (Huttl et al 2005).

Actually in laparoscopic antireflux surgery there are two debated questions today: if partial or total fundusplication must be performed and if this last is preferred division of short gastric vessels must be routinely performed or not.

6.1 Partial versus total fundoplcation
The total fundoplication involves a 360-degree wrap of the gastric fundus around the esophagus and is the most commonly performed anti-reflux operation. Total wrap (Nissen) supports and acknowledge the fact that the wrap needs to be "floppy" to minimize postoperative dysphagia (DeMeester et al 1986). It should also be noted that a floppy Nissen fundoplication is safe and effective in patients suffering from a defective esophageal peristalsis. Finally, proponents of the Nissen note a decreased effectiveness of a partial Fundoplication in controlling reflux symptoms.

Series	FU (years)	N (%FU)	%Hb Relief (0-1)	Revision (%)	Off PPI+H2-A (%)
Morgenthal et al. 2007 (Emory, GA, USA)	11,0	166 (59)	89	10,8	70
Dallemagne et al. 2006 (Belgium)	10,3	45 (66)	96	1,4	92*
Kelly et al. 2007 (Australia)	10	226 (90)	84	17	79
Zaninotto et al. 2007 (Italy)	8,1	138 (95)	-	9,4	79
Bammer et al. 2001 (mayo, FL, USA)	6,4	171 (59)	94	1,0	86*
Laffularde et al. 2001 (Australia)	6	166 (93)	87	14,2	89
Oelschlager et al 2008 (Seattle, WA, USA)	5,8	288 (65)	-	3	
Anvari, Allen 2003 (Ontario, Canada)	5	181 (48)	-	3,6	88
Booth et al. 2002 (England)	4	140 (78)	90	6,3	86

FU= follow-up; HB= heartburn; 0-1= none-mild; *Does not include patients on H2-A

Table 1. Laparoscopic 360° Fundoplication Series

Two partial fundoplications are commonly performed, the Dor and Toupet fundoplication (anterior and posterior wrap). Of these two partial wraps, the Toupet is the most commonly performed partial Fundoplication (Roberts et al 2006).

The Nissen procedure finds excellent symptomatic control but is reported to also have a high postoperative dysphagia rate and specific side effects such as inability to belch and vomit, and gas bloat syndrome (Sgromo et al 2008; Watson et al 2001).

The Toupet procedure is thought to produce less postoperative side effects than the Nissen procedure but studies have indicated that the recurrence rate of reflux symptoms may be higher after this procedure (Yobe et al 1997; Fernando et al 2002).

Horvath et al defines in a study the preoperative risk factors that predispose patients to failure. Data from 48 patients with objective follow-up performed as a part of a prospective long-term outcome project: 24-h pH-monitoring, manometry, esophagogastroduodenoscopy at 6 months, 3 years and 6 years, was analyzed (Horvath et al 1999). Patients in whom testing was completed were divided into two groups based on their results: those whose procedures failed (n=22) and those who had a successful outcome after a Toupet fundoplication (n=26). Surgical failure was defined as an abnormal postoperative De Meester score, with or without symptomatic recurrence. The authors shows that age, sex, primary and secondary presenting symptoms, presence of hiatal hernia, and esophageal dysmotility were not predictive of failure following a Toupet procedure and the numbers of years of GERD symptoms before surgery also did not predict failure after Toupet fundoplication. Horvath and colleagues concluded that the laparoscopic Toupet fundoplication appears to provide a weaker antireflux barrier than the Nissen procedure and is probably an insufficient procedure for patients with severe GERD. It may also

predispose patients to postoperative mediastinal warp hernation. Independent preoperative predictors of failure after Toupet were:
- LES pressure <5mmHg an preoperative manometry,
- Distal esophageal aperistaltic segment,
- Biopsy proved Barrett's metaplasia,
- Presence of stricture,
- Grade III or IV esophagitis an endoscopy,
- Preoperative De Meester score >50.

Guerin et al in a recent randomized trial with a 3 years follow-up, compared Nissen versus Toupet Fundoplication. Both groups in this study presented comparable preoperative findings (Guerin et al 2007). The Toupet procedure presented a higher level of invaliding functional symptoms in the immediate postoperative period, and the difference with the Nissen Fundoplication group was statistically significant for hyperflautolence, solids dysphagia and incapacity to belch. But at 1 and 3 years follow-up there wasn't any statistically significant difference of invalidating symptoms and the satisfaction level remained high. The authors concluded that the choice of the technique did not seem to be determined by the preoperative investigations, except when it diagnosticated a brachy esophagus and they also confirmed that laparoscopic Nissen or Toupet Fundoplication provides a high level of patients satisfaction despite invalidating side effects during the first postoperative year.

Strate et al compared laparoscopic Toupet and Nissen Fundoplication in 200 patients with esophageal motility disorders within 2 years follow-up (Strate et al 2008). The authors led to the following conclusion:
- Esophageal motility disorder does not effect postoperative clinical outcome and requires no tailoring of surgical management;
- The Toupet procedure is more effective in reflux control;
- Postoperative dysphagia is significantly higher after Nissen Fundoplication;
- Toupet Fundoplication reduces the rate of reoperation due to mechanical failure.

For Strate and colleagues the Toupet Fundoplication seems to be the better operative procedure for patients suffering from GERD.

Another similar randomized clinical trial by Booth and colleagues compared the two procedures in 127 patients considering preoperative esophageal manometry after 1 year follow-up (Booth et al 2008). In the study there was no significant difference in the prevalence or severity of symptoms after surgery between the Nissen group and Toupet group except for a greater prevalence of dysphagia and chest pain when eating in the Nissen group and there were no postoperative differences in the prevalence or severity of symptoms between the effective and ineffective motility groups, other than an increased severity score for flatus in the effective motility group 6 months after surgery. At 1 year follow-up there were no significant differences in Visick score between Nissen and Toupet group. The authors provides no clear conclusions regarding the efficacy and durability of Nissen compared with Toupet Fundoplication in controlling the reflux symptoms of heartburn and regurgitation, although there are greater postoperative acid exposure time and more pH failures in the Toupet group.

Sgromo et al compared the long-term outcome of Nissen and Toupet fundoplication by evaluating symptoms and quality of life at 7 years follow-up (Sgromo et al 2008). The authors concluded that long-term satisfaction, general symptoms score and quality of life were equivalent after laparoscopic Nissen or Toupet fundoplication, despite, a significantly increased prevalence of persistent heartburn after laparoscopic Toupet fundoplication.

Kamolz et al used the Gastrointestinal Quality of Life Index (GIQLI) for evaluating Nissen laparoscopic fundoplication versus Toupet procedure (Kamolz et al 2002). At 3 years and 5 years follow-up, the analysis of quality of life data showed that the GIQLI score remained stable in comparison with the 1 year follow-up data. Patients satisfaction with surgery was rated as "excellent" or "good" in 97.7% of patients. There were no significant differences between the 2 groups. The authors concluded that quality of life scores for both surgical groups were almost equal and postoperative outcome were comparable to values in healthy controls.

In a similar retrospective study, Zugel et al compared the results of 122 Toupet and 40 Nissen laparoscopic fundoplication in terms of patients satisfaction at 19 months follow-up. Both groups offered effective therapy for reflux, with more than 90% patient satisfaction (Zugel et al 2002). The authors concluded that both surgical techniques were effective in the treatment of GERD.

Laws et al used a randomized prospective study to compare the Nissen fundoplication versus the Toupet fundoplication for GERD (Laws et al 1997). At 27.2 months follow-up, postoperative symptomatology was judged using a modified Visick scale using the following grades in 38 patients:

- I no symptoms,
- II minimal symptoms, no lifestyle changes, no need to see a doctor,
- III significant symptoms requiring lifestyle changes of doctor's help,
- IV debilitating symptoms or reoperation.

There were no grade IV's. At follow-up, Visick score after the Nissen wrap were I-13, II-8, III-2 and after the Toupet procedure were I-12 and II-3. The authors concluded that a partial or complete wrap after division of the short gastric vessels offers effective therapy for reflux esophagitis with >90% patients satisfaction.

Farrell and colleagues compared the effectiveness and durability of Toupet (79 pts) and Nissen (59 pts) procedures as a function of preoperative esophageal motility (Farrell et al 2000). Patients scored heartburn, regurgitation and dysphagia preoperatively, and at 6 weeks and 1 years, using 0 to 3 scale. At 6 weeks after operation, heartburn and regurgitation were similarly improved in both groups, but dysphagia was more prevalent among Nissen patients. After 1 year, heartburn and regurgitation were re-emerging in Toupet patients, and dysphagia was again similar between groups. Patients with impaired motility who have Nissen fundoplication are no more likely to suffer persistent dysphagia than their counterparts who have Toupet fundoplication. But, patients with normal motility are more likely to develop symptoms recurrence after Toupet fundoplication than Nissen procedure, with no distinction in dysphagia rates. The authors concluded that Toupet patients suffer more heartburn recurrence than Nissen patients, with similar dysphagia.

Fernando et al compared Toupet procedure versus Nissen fundoplication (Fernando et al 2002). Extended outcome and quality of life measurement (SF36 and HRQOL) were available for 142 patients at a mean follow-up of 19.7 months. Since there was a potential bias with a greater proportion of esophageal dysmotility with Toupet patients, further analysis was performed by dividing patients into four groups: group 1, Nissen patients with decreased motility; group 2, Toupet patients with decreased motility; group 3, Nissen patients with normal motility; and group 4, Toupet patients with normal motility.

Comparison were made as follows: group 1 versus group 2, group 3 versus group 4, and group decreased motility versus group normal motility. There were no significant differences between Nissen and Toupet groups except for a higher incidence of dysphagia in the Toupet group. Resumption of proton pump inhibitors was required in 20% Nissen patients compared to 38% Toupet patients (p<0.05). Only 7% in the Nissen group were dissatisfied with their surgery compared to 21% patients in the Toupet group (p<0.05). The SF36 scores were similar in all quality of life domains except for the domain of physical function, where better scores were seen in the Nissen group compared to the Toupet group (p<0.05). Comparison of group 1 versus group 2 revealed no significant difference in SF36 and HRQOL scores, symptoms, and medication use. Comparison of group 3 versus 4 demonstrated slightly worse HRQOL scores in the Toupet group and poorer scores (p<0.05) in the SF36 domains of vitality and mental health for the Toupet patients. The Toupet patients with normal motility also complained of more dysphagia and waterbrash (p<0.05). Comparison was also made between patients with impaired motility and those with normal motility. There were no differences in SF36 scores, HRQOL score, symptoms and medication use. This analysis supports the hypothesis that the differences seen were related to differences in esophageal motility. Surprisingly, they found more dysphagia in the Toupet group. These differences was not seen when they were analyzing the results of patients in the impaired motility groups but was present in patients with normal motility. The reason for this is unclear but may be related to a greater degree of recurrent esophagitis because of reflux in Toupet patients.

Dallemagne and colleagues compared laparoscopic Nissen fundoplication versus Toupet procedure at 5 years and 10 years follow-up (Dallemagne et al 2006). At 5 years follow-up, 58 Nissen patients and 28 Toupet patients completed the study, and at 10 years 49 Nissen and 20 Toupet patients completed the follow-up. At 5 years the heartburn was relieved in 98% of the Nissen group and 86% of the Toupet group. There was no significant difference between the two groups. Ten years after surgery the heartburn still was controlled in 96% of Nissen patients and 90% of Toupet group. Also in this case there was no significant difference between the two groups. Kaplan-Meier estimates of recurrence-free proportion were evaluated and control of reflux was still obtained in 93.3% of the Nissen groups and 81.8 % of Toupet patients at 10 years (p=0.17). There was no significant difference in the incidence of side effects between partial and total fundoplication. The incidence of postoperative dysphagia in patients with preoperative impaired esophageal motility was not different after partial or total fundoplication. Dallemagne and colleagues concluded that Nissen patients have better results than Toupet patients, although the differences was not statistically significant and they observed more recurrences after partial fundoplication than after Nissen fundoplication.

Fein et al compared partial fundoplication versus total fundoplication at 10 years follow-up. 88 patients received a Nissen procedure and 10 a Toupet fundoplication (Fein et al 2008). Follow-up of the patients included disease-related questionnaire and GastroIntestinal Quality of Life Index (GIQLI). Positive pH score were 21% in Nissen group and 56% in Toupet patients. The heartburn was present in 29.7% of Nissen groups and 12.5% of Toupet patients, regurgitation in 15.1% of the Nissen group and 10% of the Toupet group, dysphagia in 30.6% of the Nissen group and 28.6% of the Toupet group. Patients who had undergone Toupet fundoplication (43%) took proton pump inhibitors significantly more often than patients who underwent Nissen fundoplication (14%). None of the differences regarding the various procedures were significant about the GIQLI. In the observational scores, Nissen fundoplication appeared to control reflux better than partial fundoplication.

In conclusion, despite the difficulties in comparing the result of single experiences of partial and total placation almost all combined experiences reported a good clinical and instrumental result for Toupet and Nissen procedures with light preference of Nissen for a better reflux control with similar others side effects.

6.2 Division versus non division of the short gastric vessels

The total fundoplication wrap achieves very effective control of reflux, although it can be followed by some troublesome side effects, such as dysphagia, gas bloat and inability to belch. To minimize the risk of developing these side effects, Nissen's procedure has been modified in a variety of ways concerning the length of the placation (short: 2 cm, long: 3-4 cm), its contention's degree (tight or floppy), the fixation of posterior wrap to the diaphragm or the esophagus, the routine iatal repair and the routine division of the first two or three short gastric vessels (true, Nissen) or it's preservation (Rossetti variation). There is a general agreement in literature to prefer a short floppy placation with no routine iatal repair and no wrao fixation. A still debated question is the significance of short gastric vessels division (deMeester et al 1986). It has been claimed that this step is followed by a lower risk of dysphagia, gas bloat and other side effects (deMeester et al 1986; Donehaue et al 1985) However, some surgeons claim that an equally good outcome can be achieved without dividing these vessels (Rossetti et al 1977; Watson et al 1997; Watson et al 1995; Anvari et al 1996) and this evidence is confirmed by randomized controlled trial.

Chryos et al in a prospective randomized trial compared Nissen (with division gastric vessels) to Nissen-Rossetti (without division gastric vessels) technique after 12 months follow-up (Chryos et al 2001). The authors concluded that division of short gastric vessels while performing laparoscopic Nissen fundoplication does not improve clinical outcome and laboratory finding in patients with GERD, and, at the same time, is associated with prolongation of the operating time and increased incidence of postoperative gas bloat syndrome.

In a recent multicentric trial of 1340 patients, Pessaux et al, concluded that the division of short gastric vessels did not improve clinical outcome after 2 or 5 years follow-up and increased the incidence of gas discomfort (Pessaux et al 2005).

In a recent randomized controlled trial Yang, Watson and colleagues reported the clinical outcome at 10 years follow-up (Yang et al 2008). The surgeons of this study have just reported the 6 months and 5 years outcome from this trial in previous publications (O'Boyle et al 2002; Watson et al 1997).

The authors confirm what many other papers claim: the division of the short gastric vessels does not influence the clinical outcome (Luostarinen et al 1999; Blomqvist et al 2000).

At 10 years follow-up, the authors concluded that there were no significant differences between the 88 patients that completed the study for either incidence or severity of dysphagia, heartburn, or overall satisfaction. These outcomes were identical to the outcomes from the earlier follow-up.

In a study of 138 patients, Sato et al analyzed the effect of short gastric vessels division on postoperative dysphagia (Sato et al 2002). They reported that laparoscopic Nissen fundoplication with or without division of short gastric vessels achieved a similar outcome. Their research suggested that patient selection and accurate construction of the fundoplication were the most important factors in minimizing postoperative dysphagia.

Mardani, Lundell and colleagues designed a randomized controlled trial to determine the long-term results of total Nissen Fundoplication with or without division of short gastric vessels in a 10 years follow-up (Mardani et al 2009). They reported that mechanical side-effects remain a problem following construction of a total wrap, and are perhaps of even greater concern when the operation is performed laparoscopically. There is a widely held view among surgeons that a wrap should be short end tension free (deMeester et al 1986; Rossetti et al 1977). However, the optimal length of total wrap to minimize subsequent obstructive complaints remains to be clarified in Mardani and colleagues randomized trial, in fact it may sometimes be necessary to divide some of the short gastric vessels in order to construct a tension free wrap, but this cannot be recommended in routine surgical practice (Mardani et al 2009). In a precedent report the same authors have reported subtle manometric differences between the two study groups, offering a physiologic background to a potential difference in functional outcome (Engstrom et al 2004), but it appears that these differences in lower esophageal sphincter response to gastric distension with air do not translate into important and clinically relevant functional correlates.

At 10 years follow-up, the authors concluded that with total Fundoplication it makes no difference whether the fundus is mobilized or not and that both types of repair provide long-lasting control of reflux (Mardani et al 2009).

Leggett et al. compared laparoscopic Nissen Fundoplication and Rossetti's modification in 239 patients, follow-up for the Rossetti group (138 patients) extends from 36 to 82 months and that for the Nissen group (101 patients) from 17 to 35 months (Leggett et al 2000). All patients experienced relief from symptomatic gastroesophageal reflux, whether they received the Rossetti modification or the Nissen Fundoplication. In their series, they found no statistically significant differences in intraoperative, postoperative, or overall complications between the two procedures. Prolonged postoperative dysphagia requiring dilation was significantly higher in the Rossetti group than in the Nissen group. But the percentage of patients requiring dilatation in both groups was higher in the first 20 than in the last 20 cases, and the authors state that with experience, surgeons become better able to judge the tightness of the crural closure, the size of posterior window, and the looseness of the wrap.

Table 2 shows of results of a different series that compared total fundoplication with or without division short gastric vessels.

In another prospectively randomized trial Kosek and colleagues compared the clinical and functional results after total fundoplication with or without division of short gastric vessels after five years follow-up (Kosek et al 2009). During long-term follow-up median DeMeester score decreased without statistically significant differences between the two groups and Gastrointestinal Quality of Life and patient satisfaction were similar in both group. The authors concluded that in their patient population division of the short gastric vessels during Nissen fundoplication that it has no statistically significant influence on clinical or functional outcome during a 5-year follow-up period. They therefore do not recommend routine division of the short gastric vessels in the course of total fundoplication. The intraoperative decision to divide the vasa gastricae breves may be made in some patients to obtain a tension-free fundoplication.

Finally in spite that many authors still routinely employ Nissen technique to perform a 360 degree short fundoplication there is no evidence support this position according to randomized study.

Rossetti variation (without section of short gastric vessels) can be "short e floppy" as well according the surgeon's experience and the use of an endoesophageal bougie of 54 – 60 Fr.

	Crysos et al. – 12 months FU *		Pessaux et al. – 5 years FU *		Yang et al. – 10 years FU		Mardani et al. – 10 years FU **	
	Not Divided 32 pt	Divided 24 pt	Not Divided 404 pt	Divided 305 pt	Not divided 44 pt (%)	Divided 44 pt (%)	Not Divided 31 pt	Divided 42 pt
Reccurence	-	-	35 (8,7)	40 (13,1)	-	-	-	-
Heartburn	0	1 (4)	-	-	18	11	1,9 (1,4)	1,4 (0,7)
Chest pain	1 (3)	0	1 (0,25)	0	-	-	-	-
Regurgitation	0	0	-	-	17	9	-	-
Respiratory	2 (16)	1 (4)	2 (0,5)	2 (0,6)	20	24	-	-
Dysphagia	5 (16)	4 (17)	26 (6,4)	28 (9,2)			2,4 (1,6)	2,0 (1,5)
Solids	5	4	-	-	44	59	-	-
Liquids	0	0	-	-	14	14	-	-
Gas-bloating Syndrome	6 (19)	9 (38)	44 (10,9)	26 (8,5)	32	41	-	-
Diarrhea	-	-	3 (0,7)	7 (2,3)	-	-	2,6 (1,6)	2,4 (1,5)
Indigestion	-	-	3 (0,7)	6 (2)	-	-	3,1 (1,5)	3,4 (1,2)
Constipation	-	-	1 (0,25)	0	-	-	2,3 (1,2)	2,4 (1,3)
Abdominal pain	-	-	4 (1)	7 (2,3)	-	-	2,8 (1,4)	2,5 (1,2)
Hiccup	-	-	2 (0,5)	2 (0,6)	-	-	-	-
Flatulence	-	-	8 (2)	12 (4)	-	-	-	-
Nausea	-	-	0	1 (0,3)	10	21	-	-

Pt= patients; *=Numbers in parentheses represent percentages. **=Values are mean (s.e.m.). In all series no significant differences demonstrated between trial groups.

Table 2. Laparoscopic Total fundoplication: not divided (Nissen-Rossetti procedure) vs divided (Nissen procedure) short gastric vessels.

In the few cases in which a "floppy" placation is not feasible than short gastric vessels must be divided and there a Nissen procedure performed.

In conclusion, Laparoscopic fundoplication is an established treatment for symptomatic gastro esophageal reflux disease and must be considered now days as the "gold standard" surgical procedure, tailoring a only marginal role to open surgery. It effectively controls heartburn and regurgitation, but it can be associated with unwanted effects, principally postoperative dysphagia, postprandial fullness, inability to belch or vomit and increased passage of flatus (tab. 2).

The choice of a total (360 degree) or a partial (270 degree) placation is difficult and not supported with clear evidence both in randomized and non randomized series, even if a better control of reflux symptoms in long follow-up studies gave a reason of a much a larger experience of 360 degree plication performed by reflux surgeon.

Total fundoplication is than the most performed operation for surgical treatment of GERD. Division of short gastric vessels (Nissen) or their preservation (Rossetti variation) is the last debated point. Randomized and non-randomized studies seem to point out in a precise way that a division of short gastric vessels is unnecessary to perform a "short and floppy" placation: the two main objectives to achieve is to prevent post operative dysphagia.

7. Barrett's esophagus

Barrett's esophagus is an acquired abnormality that is characterized grossly by an upward displacement of the squamo-columnar junction, with replacement of the typical whitish smooth esophageal mucosa by a velvety, reddish mucosa (Oelschlager et al 2003). The columnar-lined esophagus was described by Norman Barrett in 1950 (Barrett 1950), reported to be associated with gastroesophageal reflux disease in 1953 (Allison et al 1953) and convincingly linked with oesophageal adenocarcinoma in 1975 (Naef et al 1975). The paradigm is that Barrett's esophagus arises as a complication of symptomatic gastroesophageal reflux disease and predisposes to esophageal adenocarcinoma.

BE is detected in approximately 6–12% of patients with GERD (Winters et al 1987, Cameron et al 1992). At present, BE is the most common cause of esophageal adenocarcinoma, a deadly malignancy with a frequency that has been rising strikingly in Western countries and a mortality rate that still exceeds 80% (Parker et 1997). In the USA, the incidence of esophageal adenocarcinoma has increased more than sixfold over the past three decades (Pohl et al 2005). The absolute risk of patients with BE for developing cancer is approximately 0.5% per year (Hirota et al 1999).

The metaplastic mucosa was confirmed by biopsy of the tubular esophagus during endoscopy.

Controversy over criteria for diagnosis of BE primarily concerns whether intestinal metaplasia (IM) is required for a diagnosis of BE. In the USA, BE has been defined by the Parameters Committee of the American College of Gastroenterology as the metaplastic replacement of any length of the esophageal epithelium that can be recognized at endoscopy and that is confirmed by biopsy to have specialized intestinal metaplasia, defined by the presence of goblet cells (Wang et al 2008). The vast majority of adenocarcinomas of the esophagus are accompanied by IM in multiple studies (Paraf et al 1995; Cameron et al 1995, Smith et al 1984). Therefore, it has been believed that esophageal adenocarcinoma arises in intestinal type mucosa with goblet cells within a columnar-lined esophagus (CLE).

CLE can involve any of three types of epithelium: fundic (gastric), cardial (junctional), and specialized intestinal metaplasia.

The British Society of Gastroenterology does not require confirmation of intestinal metaplasia in biopsies from the esophagus to establish this diagnosis (Gastroenterology TBSO 2005; Playford et al 2006.

In the concept of these guidelines, the presence of IM is thought to be less important for the diagnosis of BE than the presence of a proper esophageal gland, squamous island, and/or double muscularis mucosa (Takubo et al 1991; Takubo et al 1995; Long et al 1999). The most important rationale behind this view is related to the high rate of sampling errors at index endoscopy. Repeated endoscopy and biopsy are often necessary to confidently detect or exclude the presence of IM. Based on a recent retrospective study, an estimated eight biopsies are necessary for an adequate assessment of the presence of intestinal metaplasia (Harrison et al 2007). Furthermore, a previous study from the UK National Barrett's Oesophagus Registry (UKBOR) has not only confirmed this, but has demonstrated a similar neoplastic risk in patients with columnar metaplasia with and without demonstrable intestinal metaplasia (Vaezi et al 1996; Lieberman et al 1997; Locke et 2003; Smpliner et al

2002; Watson et al 2005; Shepherd et al 2003; Gatenby et al 2008). The relative risk of adenocarcinoma development in patients with columnar-lined esophagus has been estimated at 5–125 fold higher than of control populations (Van der Veen et al 1989; Bartelsman et al 1992; Iftikar et al 1992; Solaymani-Dodaran et 2004; Anderson et al 2003) with the overall annual adenocarcinoma risk in columnar-lined esophagus at 0.69% (range 0–3.6%) per annum (Gatenby et al 2008).

Like the British Society of Gastroenterology, the Japan Esophageal Society defines BE as a CLE with at least one of the following: a proper esophageal gland, squamous island, or double muscularis mucosae (Japan esophageal Society 2009). In a recent review of 141 cases, Takubo *et al.* demonstrated that more than 70% of primary esophageal adenocarcinomas were adjacent to cardiac and/or fundic rather than intestinal type mucosa with goblet cells (Takubo et al 2009). This suggests BE might be better defined as the presence of metaplastic columnar-lined esophagus with or without goblet cells, which is in accordance with the British and Japanese definition of BE. As there are still few data on the risk of esophageal adenocarcinoma in CLE lacking IM.

Controversy has surrounded the most appropriate means of reflux control in patients with CLE. While pharmacological acid suppression is the least invasive and most suitable for elderly patients and those with comorbidity, the high incidence of hiatal hernia, lower esophageal sphincter failure, peristaltic impairment, and reflux of duodenal juice renders proton pump inhibitor (PPI) therapy less effective in columnar-lined esophagus than in less severe reflux disease, with up to 40% still demonstrating pathological acid exposure after receiving up to 80 mg per day of omeprazole (Lundell et al 2001; Katzka et al 1994; Sampliner et al 1994; Ouatu-Lascar et al 1998; Sharma et al 1997). Several series have suggested that fundoplication, by virtue of its ability to correct hiatal hernia, lower esophageal sphincter failure, and reflux of duodenal juice, confers some protection against adenocarcinoma development (Wassnaar et al 2010).

In conclusion BE and CLE may be considered as a synonym.

Progression of BE in this paper is defined as a change in histological findings on biopsy from CLE to any form of dysplasia or an increase in grade of dysplasia. Development of adenocarcinoma is also considered progression of disease. Regression is defined as change from high-grade dysplasia (HGD) to low-grade dysplasia (LGD) or no dysplasia, change from LGD to metaplasia or loss of metaplasia, and change from CLE to complete loss of metaplasia. Shortening of the segment or development of squamous cell islands, although considered by some as regression, usually is not accurately measured and reported, and is therefore, not considered regression in our report. Long-segment BE (LSBE) is defined as > 3 cm, short segment BE (SSBE) is defined as a length 1- 3 cm seen at endoscopy and confirmed by biopsy, ultra-short segment Barrett Esophagus < 1cm.

The goal of treatment of columnar-lined esophagus is to prevent non-neoplastic complications and development of dysplasia and adenocarcinoma by control of gastroesophageal reflux while maintaining a healed mucosa (Sampliner et al 2002).

Patients with columnar-lined esophagus are among those with the most severe gastroesophageal reflux disease (Winters et al 1987; Avidan et al 2002; Liebermann et al 1997; Locke et al 2003, Csendes et al 2002) and adequate control of reflux is difficult (Katzka et al 1994; Ouatu-Lascar et al 1998; Sharma et al 1997). Medical therapy does not prevent biliary reflux into the esophagus (Vaezi et 1996; Manifold et al 2000), and only surgical correction of the defective gastroesophageal sphincter can abolish this (Parilla et al 2003; Watson et al 1997; Zaninotto et al 2002).

Three recent studies have investigated the effect of PPI treatment on the risk of progression of BE to dysplasia or adenocarcinoma (Cooper et al 2006; Hillman et al 2004; Nguyen et al 2009). The results of these controlled studies suggest a protective effect of PPIs in limiting the progression of BE, but they do not eliminate the risk of developing AC.

In the study by Hillman et al, patients were stratified according to delay in starting PPI therapy after the diagnosis of BE was established (Hillman et al 2004). Patients who delayed PPI therapy for ≥ 2 years after being diagnosed with BE had 5.6 times higher risk of developing low grade dysplasia than patients who used PPI within the first year after diagnosis. Furthermore, patients with BE had up to a 20 times higher risk of developing high grade dysplasia or adenocarcinoma when PPI therapy was delayed for 2 years after diagnosis of BE. Although this suggests a substantial protective effect, the absolute risk of developing high grade dysplasia or adenocarcinoma was low, 3%, at a median follow-up of 4.7 years. The small rate of progression of BE makes it very difficult to show a difference between treatments.

In another study, Cooper et al considered 188 patients with IM who were treated with a PPI, the risk of developing low grade dysplasia within 5 years of the diagnosis of BE was around 2.5%, and the risk of high grade dysplasia or adenocarcinoma was around 2% while taking PPI therapy (Cooper et al 2006).

However, when following patients for > 5 years, Nguyen et al recently have found a much higher risk of developing adenocarcinoma (Nguyen et al 2009). They have studied 344 patients diagnosed with BE without dysplasia, with a mean follow-up of 7.6 years. They found that the chance of developing HGD or adenocarcinoma was 7.4%. Moreover, this risk was even higher when not taking PPIs (14.2%).

The hypothesis that surgery is superior to medical therapy comes from the assumption that surgery provides better control of GERD than do PPIs, and this should translate into lower progression rates. There have been very few studies comparing medical and surgical therapy.

Gatenby et al published the results of their review of a cohort of 738 patients with BE (Gatenby et al 2009). They compared 41 patients with anti-reflux surgery to 551 treated medically with PPIs, 42 patients treated with H2 receptor antagonists (H2RAs), 95 patients treated with H2RA followed by PPI and 9 patients with treatment. After a follow-up of 5 years after medical therapy and 6 years after surgical therapy, there was however a trend toward antireflux surgery being more protective. No patients in the antireflux group developed HGD or AC as compared to 4.3% in the all-medical therapies group (P = 0.13). There were not enough patients in the surgical arm to determine if this was a significant difference.

Parrilla et al have published the only randomized study comparing 43 patient treated with medical treatment and 58 with antireflux surgery (Parrilla et al 2003). In that study, 101 patients with BE were treated between 1982 and 2000. Medical treatment consisted of H2RA treatment initially and then omeprazole from 1992 onward. Surgery was performed through laparotomy with Nissen fundoplication in 56 patients and a Collis-Nissen procedure in the other two because of short esophagus. All patients had annual clinical, endoscopic and histological follow-up, and patients who had an operation also had a pH study and manometry at 1 year postoperatively and every 5 years thereafter, or if they presented with recurrent GERD symptoms. Mean follow-up was 6 years for the medical therapy group and 7 years for the surgical group. Progression of BE to any dysplasia was found in eight patients (19%) in the medical treatment group and in three in the surgical group (5%). Two patients in each group progressed to adenocarcinoma, which was confirmed after esophageal resection. Although differences in progression rates between the two groups were not significant according to the authors, when a sub-analysis was performed including only patients in the surgical arm with normal pH, the progression rate dropped to 2%, which was a significantly lower chance of progression of disease than in the medical group.

The hypothesis that surgery is superior to medical therapy comes from the assumption that surgery provides better control of GERD than do PPIs, and this should translate into lower progression rates. The control of reflux is essential in preventing progression of disease, is backed up by the fact that, in most studies, the patients with progression after surgical treatment seem to have recurrent reflux. This observation, that control of reflux is essential in preventing progression of disease, is backed up by the fact that, in most studies, the patients with progression after surgical treatment seem to have recurrent reflux (Oelschlager et al 2003; O'Riordan et al 2004; Biertho et al 2007; Lagergren et al 2007; Csendes et al 2004).

Hofstetter et al have published the study with the longest follow-up (Hofstetter et al 2001). They showed results for a series of 97 patients, with complete endoscopic follow-up in 79, at a median of 5 years. No patients developed HGD or adenocarcinoma, but four had progression of metaplasia to LGD (5%).

Bowers et al, have reported a similar series with a mean follow-up of 4.6 years (Bowers et al 2002). Their 104 patients underwent open or laparoscopic fundoplication. Of these, 64 patients had endoscopic follow-up with biopsy. None of the patients developed HGD or adenocarcinoma. Only one patient had progression to LGD (1.5%).

Wassenaar and Oelschlager in a recent review are summarized the result of 11 publications on surgical treatment for BE that included results on prevention of progression, as well as regression of metaplasia or dysplasia (Wassenaar et al 2010). A total of 551 patients were considered with a median follow up of 3.6 years. The progression rate of metaplasia to dysplasia or adenocarcinoma was 3.4% and 0.7% respectively and the regression rate was 30.5%.

Kamolz and colleagues evaluated and compared quality of life data before and after laparoscopic antireflux surgery in GERD patients with and without BE (Kamolz et al 2003). The authors concluded that non-BE patients undergoing laparoscopic antireflux surgery achieved a better quality of life improvement than those patients with BE. The authors compared QoL data of both groups to the mean value of general population. This means that laparoscopic antireflux surgery is able to improve QoL significantly in all GERD patients, with and without BE.

In Conclusion, surgical treatment is able only to control acid and biliopancreatic refluxate, with an improvement of quality of life. A very important point of view is the efficacy of antireflux barrier, infact after surgical treatment, there is also still progression of disease although the risk seems to become very small when this treatment is successful.

The complexity of assessment and management of CLE require a multidisciplinary approach, in regard of diagnosis and strategies of treatment. This is particularly true for surgical therapy, which has to be effective and long lasting; therefore, it should be preferably performed by experienced surgical teams.

8. Quality of life after antireflux surgery

The large success of laparoscopic surgery as an effective treatment of gastroesophageal reflux disease, has established minimal invasive surgery as the gold standard in surgical treatment of this condition. Among antireflux procedures, laparoscopic total fundoplication is the most commonly used, providing excellent symptom relief (Watson et al 1996). Antireflux surgery has been shown to improve not only symptoms, but also quality-of life (QoL) (Velanovich et 1999; Trus et al 1999).

Laparoscopic Nissen fundoplication constructs an antireflux barrier in the cardia region and effectively controls the typical symptoms of gastroesophageal reflux disease in approximately 85-90% (Bammer et al 2001; Beldi et al 2002; Eubancs et 2000; Carlson et al 2001) of cases at 5 to 10 years follow-up and has low morbidity and mortality rates.

Poor surgical results are caused by mechanical problems or persistence of symptoms (Campos et al 1999; Rice et al 2000).

A proportion of patients have persistent reflux symptoms and require use of proton pump inhibitors despite normal functional studies (Eubancs et al 2000; Khajanchee et al 2002; Galvani et al 2003).

In our study only 5.9% required PPI post-operatively and the satisfaction rate was 63.8% at 6 months and 83.3% at 12 months, with a Johnson&DeMeester score of 8.05 (IQR: 6.95-10.20) at 6 months and to 7.60 (IQR: 7.60-9.50) at the 12 months follow-up.

After antireflux surgery we observed a significant reduction in both severity and frequency scores of heartburn, epigastric pain, regurgitation, and respiratory symptoms, but an increase of dysphagia for solids and/or liquids. This point of view may affect the improvement of quality of life after Nissen-Rossetti fundoplication. The dysphagia was reported especially during the first 3 postoperative months, and in most cases it could be controlled by diet modifications as it gradually subsided (Loustarinen et al 2001; Mungan et al 1999; Balci et al 2007).

In our series we observed 19.4% of dysphagia for solids and/or liquids at 1 months postoperatively and only 2 readmissions, with need for endoscopic ballon dilatation in one case, but at 3 months all symptoms had disappeared.

Trus et al reported a significant and durable improvement in all 8 scales of the SF-36 at 6 weeks and 1 year after laparoscopic antireflux surgery (Trus et al 1999).

Amato et al reported that dysphagia for solids and/or liquids was the only significant symptom associated with 3 of 8 scales (physical function, role physical and bodily pain) (Amato et al 2008). A border line association was found between bloating and other 3 of 8 scales (social function, role-emotional and mental health).

Peters et al found no improvement in all 8 scales, with the exception of bodily pain, in 46 patients at a median of 21 months after laparoscopic Nissen fundoplication (Peters et al 1998).

In our series we observed good results of surgical procedures with a DeMeester score after 6 months like 8.05 and after 12 months 7,60 (p< 0.0001) and an improvement of quality of life measured in all subdomains of SF-36 at 6 months and 12 months.

In our series, also, we evaluated the impact of Nissen-Rossetti fundoplication with GERD-HRQL to measure the relation between symptoms and the quality of life of patients before and after surgery.

Balci et al measured QoL with SF-36 and GERD-HRQL in 60 patients at 1 months and 6 months which showed that QoL increased significantly for all their patients after surgery (Balci et al 2007).

In all subdomains of the SF-36 the patients score increased, showing an improved quality of life in the related aspects of each item and the GERD-HRQL score showed a corresponding increase.

In another study Velanovich compared SF-36 and GERD-HRQL (Velanovich 1998). In that study, multivariate analysis showed that the only significant predictor of patient satisfaction was GERD-HRQL.

Several studies have suggested an influence of psychopathological disorders on the results of laparoscopic fundoplication (Watson et al 1997; Velanovich 2006). Kamolz et al compared the postoperative results of laparoscopic fundoplication in 21 patients with anxiety disorders diagnosed with the International Classification of Diseases 10 (ICD-1) and 21 controls. Although patients with anxiety disorders showed improvements in both their clinical parameters and the postoperative quality of life using the GIQLI questionnaire, such improvements were lower than those seen in control subjects. However, authors stated that these patients should not be excluded from surgery, and that an improvement in panic attacks was seen in one-third of them (Kamolz et al 2001).

These same authors conducted a similar case–control study on 38 patients diagnosed with major depression according to the ICD-10 classification and found that, despite adequate preoperative selection and normalization of functional parameters, these patients showed less symptomatic relief and poorer results in the postoperative GIQLI quality-of-life questionnaire as compared with control cases (Kamolz et al 2003). The same group documented improvement of results and quality of life in patients undergoing surgery for GERD with stress-related symptoms depending on whether or not they had also received psychological therapy (Kamolz et al 2001).

In our study all patients after surgery presented an improvement in quality of life measured by GERD-HRQL, with 25 (IQR 10-35.5) preoperatively, and 7 (IQR 3.5-10.15) at 6 months, and 5 (IQR 2.5-9.5) at 12 months.

In conclusion laparoscopic Nissen-Rossetti fundoplication is a safe and effective surgical procedure for treatment of GERD, generally offering an improvement of quality of life.

Finally, all patients of this series experienced an improvement in their postoperative quality of life.

9. References

Allison PR & Johnstone AS (1953). The oesophagus lined with gastric mucous membrane. Thorax;8:87–101.

Amato G, Limongelli P, Pascariello A, Rossetti G, Del Genio G, Del Genio A et al (2008). Association between persistent symptoms and long-term quality of life after laparoscopic total fundoplication. Am J Sur; 196: 582-586.

Anderson LA, Murray LJ, Murphy S J et al(2003). Mortality in Barrett's oesophagus: results from a population based study. Gut; 52: 1081–1084.

Anvari M & Allen C (2003). Five-year comprehensive outcomes evaluation in 181 patients after laparoscopic Nissen fundoplication. J Am Coll Surg.;196:51-57

Anvari M & Allen CJ (1996). Prospective evaluation of dysphagia before and after laparoscopic Nissen fundoplication without routine division of short gastrics. Surg Laparosc Endosc.;6:424-429.

Attwood SE, Lundell L, Ell C, Galmiche JP, Hatlebakk J, Fiocca R, Lind T, Eklund S, Junghard O; The LOTUS Trial Group (2008). Standardization of Surgical Technique in Antireflux Surgery: The LOTUS Trial Experience. World J Surg.;32:995-998.

Avidan B, Sonnenberg A, Schnell T G, Chejfec G, Metz A & Sontag S J (2002). Hiatal hernia size, Barrett's length and severity of acid reflux are all risk factors for oesophageal adenocarcinoma. Am J Gastroenterol; 97: 1930–1936.

Bajbouj M, Becker V, Neuber M, et al (2007). Combined pH-metry/impedance monitoring increases the diagnostic yield in patients with atypical gastroesophageal reflux symptoms. Digestion;76(3 4):223–8.

Balci D & Turkcapar AG (2007). Assessment of Quality of Life after Laparoscopic Nissen Fundoplication in Patients with Gastroesophageal Reflux Disease, World J Surg; 31: 116-121.

Bammer T, Hinder RA, Klaus A & Klingler PJ (2001). Five- to eight-year outcome of the first laparoscopic Nissen fundoplications. J Gastrointest Surg.;5:42-48.

Barham CP, Gotley DC,Mills A & Alderson D (1995). Precipitating causes of acid reflux episodes in ambulant patients with gastro-oesophageal reflux disease. Gut;36:505–10.

Barrett N (1950). Chronic peptic ulcer of the oesophagus and 'oesophagitis'. Br. J. Surg.;38:175–182.

Bartelsman JFWM, Hameeteman W & Tytgat GN (1992). Barrett's oesophagus. Eur J Cancer Prev; 1: 323–325.

Beldi G & Glattli A. (2002) Long-term gastrointestinal symptoms after laparoscopic Nissen fundoplication. Surg Laparosc Endosc Percutan Tech;12:316-319.

Biertho L, Dallemagne B, Dewandre JM, Jehaes C, Markiewicz S, Monami B, Wahlen C &Weerts J. (2007) Laparoscopic treatment of Barrett's esophagus: long-term results. Surg Endosc; 21: 11-15.

Blomqvist A, Dalenbäck J, Hagedorn C, Lönroth H, Hyltander A & Lundell L. (2000) Impact of complete gastric fundus mobilization on outcome after laparoscopic total fundoplication. J Gastrointest Surg.;4:493-500.

Bloom S.; McCartney S. & Langmead L. (2009) The modern investigation and management of gastro-oesophageal reflux disease (GORD). Clinical Medicine, 9, 6: 600-4.

Bonatti H, Achem SR & Hinder RA. (2008) Impact of changing epidemiology of gastroesophageal reflux disease on its diagnosis and treatment. J Gastrointest Surg.;12:373-381.

Booth MI, Jones L, Stratford J & Dehn TC. (2002)Results of laparoscopic Nissen fundoplication at 2-8 years after surgery. Br J Surg.;89:476-481.

Booth MI, Stratford J, Jones L & Dehn TC (2008). Randomized clinical trial of laparoscopic total (Nissen) versus posterior partial (Toupet) fundoplication for gastro-oesophageal reflux disease based on preoperative oesophageal manometry. Br J Surg.;95:57-63.

Bowers SP, Mattar SG, Smith CD, Waring JP & Hunter JG. (2002) Clinical and histologic follow-up after antireflux surgery for Barrett's esophagus. J Gastrointest Surg; 6: 532-538.

Cameron AJ, Lomboy CT, Pera M & Carpenter HA (1995). Adenocarcinoma of the esophagogastric junction and Barrett's esophagus. Gastroenterology; 109: 1541–1546.

Cameron AJ & Lomboy CT (1992). Barrett's esophagus: Age, prevalence, and extent of columnar epithelium. Gastroenterology;103:1241–1245.

Campos GM, Peters JH, DeMeester TR, Oberg S, Crookes PF, Tan S et al (1999). Multivariate analysis of factors predicting outcome after laparoscopic Nissen fundoplication. J Gastrointest Surg; 3:292-300

Carlson MA & Frantzides CT (2001). Complications and results of primary minimally invasive antireflux procedures: a review of 10735 reported cases. J Am Coll Surg; 193: 428-39.

Catarci M, Gentileschi P, Papi C, Carrara A , Marrese R, Gaspari AL & Grassi GB (2004). Evidence-based appraisal of antireflux fundoplication. Ann Surg; 239 :325-337.

Chang E Y, Morris C D, Seltman A K, O'Rourke R W, Chan B K, Hunter J G & Jobe B A (2007) The effect of antireflux surgery on esophageal carcinogenesis in patients with barrett esophagus: a systematic review. AnnSurg 246:11-21

Chrysos E, Tzortzinis A, Tsiaoussis J, Athanasakis H, Vasssilakis J & Xynos E (2001). Prospective randomized trial comparing Nissen to Nissen-Rossetti technique for laparoscopic fundoplication. Am J Surg.;182:215-221.

Cooper BT, Chapman W, Neumann CS & Gearty JC (2006). Continuous treatment of Barrett's oesophagus patients with proton pump inhibitors up to 13 years: observations on regression and cancer incidence. Aliment Pharmacol Ther; 23:727-733

Csendes A, Burdiles P, Braghetto I & Korn O (2004). Adenocarcinoma appearing very late after antireflux surgery for Barrett's esophagus: long-term follow-up, review of the literature, and addition of six patients. J Gastrointest Surg; 8: 434-441.

Csendes A, Smok G, Quiroz J et al (2002). Functional studies in 408 patients with Barrett's esophagus, compared to 174 cases with intestinal metaplasia of the cardia. Am J Gastroenterol;97: 554–560.

Dallemagne B, Weerst JM, Jehaes C, Markiewicz S & Lombard R (1991). Laparoscopic Nissen Fundoplication: preliminary report. Surg Laparosc Endosc; 1: 138-143.

Dallemagne B, Weerts J, Markiewicz S, Dewandre JM, Wahlen C, Monami B & Jehaes C (2006). Clinical results of laparoscopic fundoplication at ten years after surgery. Surg Endosc.;20:159-165.

DeMeester TR, Bonavina L & Albertucci M (1986). Nissen fundoplication for gastroesophageal reflux disease. Evaluation of primary repair in 100 consecutive patients. Ann Surg.;204:9-20.

Dent J, El-Serag HB, Wallander MA & Johansson S (2005). Epidemiology of gastro-oesophageal reflux disease: a systematic review. Gut.;54:710-717.

Dodds WJ, Dent J, Hogan WJ et al (1982). Mechanisms of gastroesophageal reflux in patients with reflux esophagitis. N Engl J Med;307:1547–52.

Donahue PE, Samelson S, Nyhus LM & Bombeck CT (1985). The floppy Nissen fundoplication. Effective long-term control of pathologic reflux. Arch Surg.;120:663-668.

Engström C, Blomqvist A, Dalenbäck J, Lönroth H, Ruth M & Lundell L (2004). Mechanical consequences of short gastric vessel division at the time of laparoscopic total fundoplication. J Gastrointest Surg.;8:442-447.

Eubanks TR, Omelanczuk P, Richards C, Pohl D & Pellegrini CA (2000). Outcomes of laparoscopic antireflux procedures. Am J Surg; 179: 391-5.

Farrell TM, Archer SB, Galloway KD, Branum GD, Smith CD & Hunter JG (2000). Heartburn is more likely to recur after Toupet fundoplication than Nissen fundoplication. Am Surg.;66:229-236.

Fass R, Quan SF, O'Connor GT, Ervin A & Iber C (2005). Predictors of heartburn during sleep in a large prospective cohort study. Chest;127:1658-66.

Fein M, Bueter M, Thalheimer A, Pachmayr V, Heimbucher J, Freys SM & Fuchs KH (2008). Ten-year outcome of laparoscopic antireflux surgery. J Gastrointest Surg.;12:1893-1899.

Fernando HC, Luketich JD, Christie NA, Ikramuddin S & Schauer PR (2002). Outcomes of laparoscopic Toupet compared to laparoscopic Nissen fundoplication. Surg Endosc.;16:905-8.

Fornari F & Sifrim D (2007). Gastroesophageal reflux and atypical symptoms: the role of impedance-pH monitoring. Digestion;76(3-4):221-2.

Galvani C, Fisichella PM, Gorodner MV, Perretta S & Patti MG (2003). symptoms are a poor indicator of reflux status after fundoplication for gastroesophageal reflux disease. Role of esophageal functions test. Arch Surg; 138:514-9

Gastroenterology TBSO (2005). Guidelines for the diagnosis and management of Barrett's columnar-lined oesophagus . cited; Available from: http://www.bsg.org.uk.

Gatenby PA, Caygill CPJ, Ramus JR, Charlett A & Watson A (2008). Barrett's columnar-lined oesophagus: demographic associations and adenocarcinoma risk. Dig Dis Sci; 53: 1175-1185.

Gatenby PA, Ramus JR, Caygill CPJ, Shepherd NA, Watson A (2008). The relevance of detection of intestinal metaplasia in columnar-lined esophagus. Scand J Gastroenterol;43:524-530.

Gatenby PA, Ramus JR, Caygill CP, Charlett A, Winslet MC & Watson A (2009). Treatment modality and risk of development of dysplasia and adenocarcinoma in columnar-lined esophagus. Dis Esophagus; 22: 133-142.

Guérin E, Bétroune K, Closset J, Mehdi A, Lefèbvre JC, Houben JJ, Gelin M, Vaneukem P & El Nakadi I (2007). Nissen versus Toupet fundoplication: results of a randomized and multicenter trial. Surg Endosc;21:1985-1990.

Hampel H, Abraham NS & El-Serag HB (2005). Meta-analysis: obesity and the risk for gastroesophageal reflux disease and its complications. Ann Intern Med;143:199-211.

Harrison R, Perry I, Haddadin W et al (2007). Detection of intestinal metaplasia in Barrett's esophagus: An observational comparator study suggests the need for a minimum of eight biopsies. Am. J. Gastroenterol.;102:1154-1161.

Hillman LC, Chiragakis L, Shadbolt B, Kaye GL & Clarke AC (2004). Proton-pump inhibitor therapy and the development of dysplasia in patients with Barrett's oesophagus. Med J Aust;180: 387-391

Hirota WK, Loughney TM, Lazas DJ, Maydonovitch CL, Rholl V & Wong RK (1999). Specialized intestinal metaplasia, dysplasia, and cancer of the esophagus and esophagogastric junction: Prevalence and clinical data. Gastroenterology;116:277–285.

Hofstetter WL, Peters JH, DeMeester TR, Hagen JA, De-Meester SR, Crookes PF, Tsai P, Banki F & Bremner CG (2001). Longterm outcome of antireflux surgery in patients with Barrett's esophagus. Ann Surg; 234: 532-538.

Horvath KD, Jobe BA, Herron DM & Swanstrom LL (1999). Laparoscopic Toupet fundoplication is an inadequate procedure for patients with severe reflux disease. J Gastrointest Surg.;3:583-591.

Hüttl TP, Hohle M, Wichmann MW, Jauch KW & Meyer G (2005). Techniques and results of laparoscopic antireflux surgery in Germany. Surg Endosc.;19:1579-87.

Iftikar SY, James PD, Steele RJC, Hardcastle JD & Atkinson M (1992). Length of Barrett's oesophagus: an important factor in the development of dysplasia and adenocarcinoma. Gut; 33:1155–1158.

Japan Esophageal Society (2009). Japanese Classification of Esophageal Cancer, tenth edition: Part I. Esophagus ;6:1–26.

Jobe BA, Wallace J, Hansen PD & Swanstrom LL (1997). Evaluation of laparoscopic Toupet fundoplication as a primary repair for all patients with medically resistant gastroesophageal reflux. Surg Endosc.;11:1080-1083.

Johnson LF (1980). 24-hour pH monitoring in the study of gastroesophageal reflux. *J Clin Gastroenterol*;2:387.

Jones RH, Hungrin ADS & Phillips J (1995). Gastroesophageal reflux disease in primary care in Europe: clinical presentation and endoscopic findings. *Eur J Gen Pract*;1:149–54.

Kahrilas PJ, Dodds WJ, Hogan WJ *et al (1986).* Esophageal peristaltic dysfunction in peptic esophagitis. *Gastroenterology*;91:897–904.

Kahrilas PJ, Dodds WJ, Hogan WJ *et al (1986).* Esophageal peristaltic dysfunction in peptic esophagitis. *Gastroenterology*;91:897–904.

Kalmoz T, Bammer T, Granderath FA & Pointer R (2001). Laparoscopic antireflux surgery in gastroesophageal reflux disease patients with concomitant anxiety disorders. Dig Liver Dis; 33: 659-664.

Kalmoz T, Granderath FA, Bammer T, Pasiut M (2001) Pointner R. Psycological intervention influences the outcome of laparoscopic antireflux surgery in patients with stress-related symptoms of gastroesophageal reflux disease. Scand J Gastroenterol ; 36: 800-805.

Kalmoz T, Granderath FA & Pointner R (2003). Does major depression in patients with gastroesophageal reflux affects the outcome of laparoscopic antireflux surgery? Surg Endosc; 17:55-60.

Kamolz T, Granderath F & Pointner R (2003). Laparoscopic antireflux surgery: disease-related quality of life assessment before and after surgery in GERD patients with and without Barrett's esophagus. Surg Endosc.;17:880-885.

Kamolz T, Granderath FA, Bammer T, Wykypiel H Jr & Pointner R (2002). "Floppy" Nissen vs. Toupet laparoscopic fundoplication: quality of life assessment in a 5-year follow-up (part 2). Endoscopy.;34:917-922.

Katzka D A & Castell D O (1994). Successful elimination of reflux symptoms does not insure adequate control of acid reflux in patients with Barrett's esophagus. Am J Gastroenterol; 89:989–991.

Kelly JJ, Watson DI, Chin KF, Devitt PG & Game PA (2007) Jamieson GG. Laparoscopic Nissen fundoplication: clinical outcomes at 10 years. J Am Coll Surg.;205:570-575.

Khajanchee YS. O'Rourke RW, Lockhart B, Patterson EJ, Hansen PD & Swanstrom LL (2002). Postopearive symptoms and failure after antireflux surgery. Arch Surg;137:1008-14.

Kösek V, Wykypiel H, Weiss H, Höller E, Wetscher G, Margreiter R & Klaus A (2009). Division of the short gastric vessels during laparoscopic Nissen fundoplication: clinical and functional outcome during long-term follow-up in a prospectively randomized trial. Surg Endosc. Oct;23:2208-13.

Laffullarde T, Watson DI, Jamieson GG, Myers JC, Game PA & Devitt PG (2001). Laparoscopic Nissen Fundoplication: five-year results and beyond. Arch Surg; 136: 180-184.

Lagergren J, Bergstrom R, Lindgren A & Nyren O (1999) Symptomatic gastroesophageal reflux as a risk factor for esophageal adenocarcinoma. N Engl J Med 340:825-831

Lagergren J & Viklund P (2007). Is esophageal adenocarcinoma occurring late after antireflux surgery due to persistent postoperative reflux? World J Surg; 31: 465-469

Laws HL, Clements RH & Swillie CM (1997). A randomized, prospective comparison of the Nissen fundoplication versus the Toupet fundoplication for gastroesophageal reflux disease. Ann Surg.;225:647-653.

Leggett PL, Bissell CD, Churchman-Winn R & Ahn C (2000). A comparison of laparoscopic Nissen fundoplication and Rossetti's modification in 239 patients. Surg Endosc.;14:473-477.

Lieberman D A, Oehlke M, Helfand M & the GORGE Consortium (1997). Risk factors for Barrett's esophagus in community-based practice. Am J Gastroenterol; 92:1293–1297.

Locke G R, Zinsmeister A R & Talley N J (2003). Can symptoms predict endoscopic findings in GERD? Gastrointest Endosc; 58: 661–670.

Long JD & Orlando RC (1999). Esophageal submucosal glands: Structure and function. Am. J. Gastroenterol.;94:2818–2824.

Loustarinen M, Vurtanen J, Koskinen M, Matikainen M & Isolauri J (2001). Dysphagia and oesophageal clearance after laparoscopic versus open Nissen fundoplication. A randomized, prospective trial. Scand J Gastroenterol;36:565-571.

Loustarinen ME & Isolauri JO (1999). Randomized trial to study the effect of fundic mobilization on long-term results of Nissen fundoplication. Br J Surg.;86:614-618.

Lundell L, Miettinen P, Myrvold HE, Hatlebakk JG, Wallin L, Malm A, Sutherland I, Walan A & Nordic GORD Study Group (2007). Seven-year follow-up of a randomized clinical trial comparing proton-pump inhibition with surgical therapy for reflux oesophagitis Br J Surg.;94:198-203.

Lundell L, Miettinen P, Myrvold HE, Pederson SA, Liedman B, Hatlebakk JG, Julkonen R, Levander K, Carlsson J, Lamm M & Wiklund I (2001). Continued (5-year) follow-up of a randomized clinical study comparing antireflux surgery and omeprazole in gastroesophageal reflux disease. J Am Coll Surg ; 192: 172-179; discussion 179:181.

Manifold D K, Marshall R E K, Anggiansah A & Owen W J (2000). Effect of omeprazole on antral duodenogastric reflux in Barrett oesophagus. Scand J Gastroenterol; 8: 796–801.

Mardani J, Lundell L, Lönroth H, Dalenbäck J & Engström C (2009). Ten-year results of a randomized clinical trial of laparoscopic total fundoplication with or without division of the short gastric vessels. Br J Surg.;96:61-65.

McKenzie D, Grayson T & Polk HC Jr (1996). The impact of omeprazole and laparoscopy upon hiatal hernia and reflux esophagitis. J Am Coll Surg; 183: 413-418.

Morgenthal CB, Shane MD, Stival A, Gletsu N, Milam G, Swafford V, Hunter JG & Smith CD (2007). The durability of laparoscopic Nissen fundoplication: 11-year outcomes. J Gastrointest Surg.;11:693-700.

Mungan Z, Demir K, Onuk MD, Göral V, Boztaş G, Beşışık F al (1999). Characteristics of gastroesophageal reflux disease in our country. Turk J Gastroenterol;10:101-106.

Naef AP, Savary M & Ozzello L (1975). Columnar-lined lower esophagus: an acquired lesion with malignant predisposition. Report on 140 cases of Barrett's esophagus with 12 adenocarcinomas. J. Thorac. Cardiovasc. Surg.;70:826-835.

Nguyen DM, El-Serag HB, Henderson L, Stein D, Bhattacharyya A & Sampliner RE (2009). Medication usage and the risk of neoplasia in patients with Barrett's esophagus. Clin Gastroenterol Hepatol; 7: 1299-1304.

O'Boyle CJ, Watson DI, Jamieson GG, Myers JC, Game PA & Devitt PG (2002). Division of short gastric vessels at laparoscopic nissen fundoplication: a prospective double-blind randomized trial with 5-year follow-up. Ann Surg;235:165-170.

Oelschlager B K, Eubanks T R, Oleynikov D, Pope C & Pellegrini C A (2002) Symptomatic and physiologic outcomes after operative treatment for extraesophageal reflux. Surg Endosc 16:1032-1036

Oelschlager BK, Barreca M, Chang L, Oleynikov D & Pellegrini CA (2003). Clinical and pathologic response of Barrett's esophagus to laparoscopic antireflux surgery. Ann Surg; 238: 458-464.

Oelschlager BK, Quiroga E, Parra JD, Cahill M, Polissar N & Pellegrini C A (2008). Long-term outcomes after laparoscopic antireflux surgery. Am J Gastroenterol.;103:280-287.

O'Riordan JM, Byrne PJ, Ravi N, Keeling PW & Reynolds JV (2004). Long-term clinical and pathologic response of Barrett's esophagus after antireflux surgery. Am J Surg; 188: 27-33.

Ouatu-Lascar R & Triadafilopoulos G (1998). Complete elimination of reflux symptoms does not guarantee normalisation of intraesophageal acid reflux in patients with Barrett's esophagus. Am J Gastroenterol; 93: 711-716.

Pandolfino JE, El-Serag HB, Zhang Q et al (2006). Obesity: a challenge to esophagogastric junction integrity. Gastroenterology;130:639-49.

Pandolfino JE, Shi G, Trueworthy B & Kahrilas PJ (2003). Esophagogastric junction opening during relaxation distinguishes nonhernia reflux patients, hernia patients, and normal subjects. Gastroenterology;125:1018-24

Paraf F, Flejou JF, Pignon JP, Fekete F & Potet F (1995). Surgical pathology of adenocarcinoma arising in Barrett's esophagus. Analysis of 67 cases. Am. J. Surg. Pathol.;19:183-191.

Parker SL, Tong T, Bolden S & Wingo PA (1997). Cancer statistics, 1997. CA Cancer J. Clin.;47:5-27.

Parrilla P, Martínez de Haro LF, Ortiz A, Munitiz V, Molina J, Bermejo J & Canteras M (2003). Long-term results of a randomized prospective study comparing medical and surgical treatment of Barrett's esophagus. Ann Surg; 237: 291-298.

Pessaux P, Arnaud JP, Delattre JF, Meyer C, Baulieux J & Mosnier H (2005). Laparoscopic antireflux surgery: five-year results and beyond in 1340 patients. Arch Surg.;140:946-951.

Peters JH, DeMeester TR, Crookes P, Oberg S, de Vos Shoop M, Hagen JA et al (1998). The treatment of gastroesophageal reflux disease with laparoscopic Nissen fundoplication: prospective evaluation of 100 patients with "typical" symptoms. Ann Surg;228:40-50.

Peters MJ, Mukhtar A, Yunus RM, Khan S, Pappalardo J, Memon B & Memon MA (2009). Meta-analysis of randomized clinical trials comparing open and laparoscopic anti-reflux surgery. Am J Gastroenterol;104:1548-61.

Playford RJ (2006). New British Society of Gastroenterology (BSG) guidelines for the diagnosis and management of Barrett's oesophagus . Gut; 55:442.

Pohl H & Welch HG (2005). The role of overdiagnosis and reclassification in the marked increase of esophageal adenocarcinoma incidence. J. Natl. Cancer Inst.; 97:142–146.

Rakita S, Villadolid D, Thomas A, Bloomston M, Albrink M, Goldin S & Rosemurgy A (2006) Laparoscopic Nissen fundoplication offers high patient satisfaction with relief of extraesophageal symptoms of gastroesophageal reflux disease. Am Surg 72:207-212.

Rice T W (2000). Why antireflux surgery fails? Dig Dis;18:43-7.

Rice T. W. & Blackstone E. H (2008). Surgical Management of Gastroesophageal Reflux Disease Gastroenterol Clin N Am 37: 901–919.

Roberts KE, Duffy AJ & Bell RL (2006). Controversies in the treatment of gastroesophageal reflux and achalasia. World J Gastroenterol.;12:3155-3161.

Rossetti M & Hell K (1977). Fundoplication for the treatment of gastroesophageal reflux in hiatal hernia. World J Surg.;1:439-443.

Rossi M, Barreca M, de Bortoli N, Renzi C, Santi S, Gennai A, Bellini M, Costa F, Conio M & Marchi S (2006). Efficacy of Nissen fundoplication versus medical therapy in the regression of low-grade dysplasia in patients with Barrett esophagus: a prospective study. Ann Surg 243:58-63.

Salminen PT, Hiekkanen HI, Rantala AP & Ovaska JT (2007). Comparison of long-term outcome of laparoscopic and conventional nissen fundoplication: a prospective randomized study with an 11-year follow-up. Ann Surg.;246:201-206.

Sampliner R E (1994). Effect of up to 3 years of high-dose lansoprazole on Barrett's esophagus. Am J Gastroenterol; 89:1844–1848.

Sampliner RE (2002). The Practice Parameters Committee of the American College of Gastroenterology. Updated guidelines for the diagnosis, surveillance, and therapy of Barrett's esophagus. Am J Gastroenterol.; 97:1888–95.

Sato K, Awad ZT, Filipi CJ, Selima MA, Cummings JE, Fenton SJ & Hinder RA (2002). Causes of long-term dysphagia after laparoscopic Nissen fundoplication. JSLS.;6:35-40.

Sgromo B, Irvine LA, Cuschieri A & Shimi SM (2008). Long-term comparative outcome between laparoscopic total Nissen and Toupet fundoplication: Symptomatic relief, patient satisfaction and quality of life. Surg Endosc.;22:1048-1053.

Sharma P, Sampliner R E & Camargo E (1997). Normalisation of esophageal pH with high-dose proton pump inhibitor therapy does not result in regression of Barrett's esophagus. Am J Gastroenterol.; 92:582-585.

Shepherd NA (2003). Barrett's esophagus: its pathology and neoplastic complications. Esophagus; 1:17-29.

Smith RR, Hamilton SR, Boitnott JK & Rogers EL (1984). The spectrum of carcinoma arising in Barrett's esophagus.A clinicopathologic study of 26 patients. Am. J. Surg. Pathol.;8:563-573.

Society of American Gastrointestinal and Endoscopic Surgeons (2010). Guidelines for surgical treatment of gastro-oesophageal reflux disease (GERD). Avaible at: http://www.sages.org/publication/id/22/

Solaymani-Dodaran M, Logan RFA, West J, Card T & Coupland C (2004). Risk of oesophageal cancer in Barrett's oesophagus and gastro-oesophageal reflux. Gut; 53: 1070-1074.

Spechler S J & Goyal R K (1996) The columnar-lined esophagus, intestinal metaplasia, and Norman Barrett. Gastroenterology 110:614-621

Spechler SJ, Lee E, Ahnen D, Goyal RK, Hirano I, Ramirez F, Raufman JP, Sampliner R, Shnell T, Sontag S, Vlahcevic ZR, Young R & Williford W (2001). Long-term outcome of medical and surgical therapies for gastroesophageal reflux disease: follow-up of a randomized controlled trial. JAMA; 285: 2331-2338.

Stanciu C & Bennett JR (1974). Alginate/antacid in the reduction of gastro-oessophageal reflux. *Lancet*;I:109-111.

Strate U, Emmermann A, Fibbe C, Layer P & Zornig C (2008). Laparoscopic fundoplication: Nissen versus Toupet two-year outcome of a prospective randomized study of 200 patients regarding preoperative esophageal motility. Surg Endosc.;22:21-30.

Takubo K, Aida J, Naomoto Y et al (2009). Cardiac rather than intestinal-type background in endoscopic resection specimens of minute Barrett adenocarcinoma. Hum. Pathol.;40: 65-74.

Takubo K, Nixon JM & Jass JR (1995). Ducts of esophageal glands proper and paneth cells in Barrett's esophagus: Frequency in biopsy specimens. Pathology;27:315-317.

Takubo K, Sasajima K, Yamashita K, Tanaka Y & Fujita K (1991). Double muscularis mucosae in Barrett's esophagus. Hum. Pathol.;22:1158-1161.

Trus TL, Laycock WS, Waring JP, Branum GD & Hunter JG (1999). Improvement in quality-of-life measures after laparoscopic antireflux surgery. Ann. Surg.;229:331-336.

Vaezi MF & Richter JE (1996). Role of acid and duodenogastroesophageal reflux in gastroesophageal reflux disease. Gastroenterology.; 111:1192-1199.

Vakil N, van Zanten SV, Kahrilas P, Dent J & Jones R (2006). The Montreal definition and classification of gastroesophageal reflux disease: a global evidence-based consensus. Am J Gastroenterol.;101:1900-1920.

Van der Veen AH, Blankenstein JD & van Blankenstein M (1989). Adenocarcinoma in Barrett's oesophagus: an overrated risk. Gut; 30: 14-18.

Velanovich V (1998). Comparison of generic (SF-36) versus disease specific (GERD-HRQL) quality of life scales for gastroesophageal reflux disease. J Gastrointest Surg.; 2:141-145.

Velanovich V (1999). Comparison of symptomatic and quality-of-life outcomes of laparoscopic and open antireflux surgery. Surgery.; 126:782-789.

Velanovich V (2006). Nonsurgical factors affecting symptomatic outcomes of antireflux surgery. Dis Esophagus. ;19: 1-4.

Wang KK & Sampliner RE (2008). Updated guidelines 2008 for the diagnosis, surveillance and therapy of Barrett's esophagus. Am. J. Gastroenterol.; 103:788–797.

Ware JE & Sherbourne CD (1992). The MOS 36-item short-form health survey (SF-36). I. Conceptual framework and item selection. Med Care; 30:473-83

Wassenaar EB & Oelschlager BK (2010). Effect of medical and surgical treatment of Barrett's metaplasia. World J Gastroenterol.;16:3773-3779.

Watson A, Heading RC & Shepherd NA (2005). Guidelines for the diagnosis and management of Barrett's columnar-lined oesophagus: a report of the working party of the British Society of gastroenterology. British Society of Gastroenterology.; London, UK; 1–42.

Watson D I, Pike G K, Baigrie R J et al (1997). Prospective doubleblind randomized trial of laparoscopic Nissen fundoplication with division and without division of short gastric vessels. Ann Surg.; 226: 642-652.

Watson DI, Chan AS, Myers JC & Jamieson GG (1997). Illness behaviour influences the outcome of laparoscopic antireflux surgery. J Am Coll Surg.; 184:44-48.

Watson DI & de Beaux AC (2001). Complications of laparoscopic antireflux surgery. Surg Endosc.;15:344-52.

Watson DI, Jamieson GG, Baigrie RJ, Mathew G, Devitt PG, Game PA, et al (1996). Laparoscopic surgery for gastroesophageal reflux : beyond the learning curve. Br J Surg; 83:1284-1287.

Watson DI, Jamieson GG, Devitt PG, Matthew G, Britten-Jones RE, Game PA & Williams RS (1995). Changing strategies in the performance of laparoscopic Nissen fundoplication as a result of experience with 230 operations. Surg Endosc.;9:961-6.

Watson DI, Pike GK, Baigrie RJ, Mathew G, Devitt PG, Britten-Jones R & Jamieson GG (1997). Prospective double-blind randomized trial of laparoscopic Nissen fundoplication with division and without division of short gastric vessels. Ann Surg.;226:642-652.

Winters C Jr, Spurling TJ, Chobanian SJ et al (1987). Barrett's esophagus. A prevalent, occult complication of gastroesophageal reflux disease. Gastroenterology.;92:118–124.

Yang H, Watson DI, Lally CJ, Devitt PG, Game PA & Jamieson GG (2008). Randomized trial of division versus nondivision of the short gastric vessels during laparoscopic Nissen fundoplication: 10-year outcomes. Ann Surg.;247:38-42.

Zagari RM, Fuccio L,Wallander MA et al (2008). Gastro-oesophageal reflux symptoms, oesophagitis and Barrett's oesophagus in the general opoulation: the Loiano-Monghidoro study. Gut;57:1354-9.

Zaninotto G, Portale G, Costantini M, Rizzetto C, Guirroli E, Ceolin M, Salvador R, Rampado S, Prandin O, Ruol A & Ancona E (2007). Long-term results (6-10 years) of laparoscopic fundoplication. J Gastrointest Surg.;11:1138-1145.

Zaninotto G, Portale G, Parenti A, Lanza C, Costantini M, Molena D, Ruol A, Battaglia G, Costantino M, Epifani M & Nicoletti L (2002). Role of acid and bile reflux in development of specialised intestinal metaplasia in distal oesophagus. Dig Liver Dis.;3:251-257.

Zügel N, Jung C, Bruer C, Sommer P & Breitschaft K (2002). A comparison of laparoscopic Toupet versus Nissen fundoplication in gastroesophageal reflux disease. Langenbecks Arch Surg.;386:494-498.

2

Laparoscopic One-Stage vs Endoscopic Plus Laparoscopic Management of Common Bile Duct Stones – A Prospective Randomized Study

Giuseppe P. Ferulano et al.*
*Department of Systemic Pathology General and
Miniinvasive Surgical Unit
University of Naples "Federico II"
Italy*

1. Introduction

The incidence of gallstones is rather high and is referred as approximately 13%-17% among the western population, [Bateson, 2000; Barbara et al., 1987; Everhart et al., 1999; Pixley et al., 1985]. It is well known that most of the people with gallstones are asymptomatic and often they are absolutely unaware of their presence, it is even referred that no more than 15-20% of them has the probability of suffering from a biliary colic later on [Attili et al., 1995], which, once occurred, could recur more easily causing sometime serious complications, such as pancreatitis by stone's migration and biliary obstruction, that over a 10-year period can be expected to occur in 2–3% of patients with initially silent gallbladder stones [Gracie & Ransohoff, 1982].

The incidence of common bile duct (CBD) stones has been reported as ranging between 5% to 18% of patients undergoing cholecystectomy for gallstones, and patients with symptoms suggestive of choledocholithiasis have an even higher incidence, also increasing with age [Martin et al., 2006]. Because of the continuous developing of the diagnostic and therapeutic techniques from the introduction of intra-operative cholangiography by Mirizzi in 1932, the choose of the most effective strategy in the management of the common bile duct (CBD) stones associated with gallstones is object of close discussions far from any conclusive agreement. The new diagnostic techniques as magnetic resonance cholangiography (MRC) and endoscopic ultrasound (EUS), give the opportunity to visualize the biliary tree without any invasive exploration of the ducts and share the same idea as the minimally invasive laparoscopic surgical approach. They are progressively evolving as well as the standard of care for the management of common bile duct (CBD) stones, historically performed via

* Saverio Dilillo, Michele D'Ambra, Ruggero Lionetti, Piero Di Silverio, Stefano Capasso, Domenico Pelaggi and Michele Rutigliano
Department of Systemic Pathology General and miniinvasive Surgical Unit (Prof. G.P.Ferulano) University of Naples "Federico II", Italy

laparotomy, which over the past decade-and-a-half has changed from open cholecystectomy with common bile duct exploration through intraoperative cholangiography or choledocoscopy, to the routine availability of endoscopic retrograde cholangioscopy (ERC) with endoscopic sphincterotomy (EST) for common bile duct (CBD) stone extraction performed before or after surgery, open in the past and laparoscopic from almost fifteen years, [Clayton et al., 2006]. However, endoscopic sphincterotomy for bile duct stones complains about a disappointing 8%–10% rate of long-term biliary complications including recurrent or residual ductal stones, cholangitis, stenosis of the papilla, and biliary pancreatitis [Paganini et al., 2007]. Macadam&Goodall, [2004] referred a high 28% rate of late, rather frequent symptoms related to low-grade cholangitis following papillosphincterotomy. Consequently the potential sequence of late persistent cholangitis should be regarded as a matter of concern, particularly in fertile female patients.

More recently laparoscopic exploration of the common bile duct (LCBDE) has been introduced for managing patients with suspected CBD stones, which allows the intraoperative definite diagnosis and the treatment at the same time, if necessary. As referred in the New Guidelines Address Management of Common Bile Duct Stones [Williams et al., 2008] the consequences are that "clinicians are now faced with a number of potentially valid options for managing patients with suspected CBDS".

Consequently the primary challenge in the management of common bile duct stones in association with gallstones nowadays is to select the best strategy with regard to success, morbidity and cost-effectiveness, [Clayton et al., 2006].

Endoscopy for common bile duct stones and surgery, mainly laparoscopic, for gallstones have been widely adopted as the preferred approach, because the results in terms of success rate, morbidity and mortality tend to overlap those of the whole surgical open approach for gallstones and common bile duct stones offering the undeniable advantages of being less invasive. The ultimate evolution of the association of laparoscopic cholecystectomy with endoscopic retrograde cholangioscopy (ERC) + endoscopic sphincterotomy (EST) was the rendez vous approach performed in a single stage operative procedure together by the surgical and the endoscopic teams, which has shown an overlapping outcome compared to other kinds of association between surgical and endoscopic procedures. Since it is commonly accepted that only a low rate of patients suffering from gallstones and undergoing laparoscopic cholecystecomy are likely to have bile duct stones identified, this procedure to be cost effective needs a definite preoperative diagnosis of common bile duct stones using the modern techniques of imaging such as MR and EUS, which can improve the likelihood of stones being found to over 90%, [Liu et al., 2001; Williams et al., 2008].

Nevertheless in the literature some limits concerning the use of endoscopy are referred like the number and the size of stones, the incidence of complications of ERC + EST occurring in 5%- 8% of cases, with mortality rates of 0.2% to 0.5% from more difficult procedures or the necessity of multiple sessions to clear completely the common bile duct requiring the use of expensive equipment and accessories. This strategy statistically increased the likelihood of complications as two or more procedures sometime should be performed in a patient to clear up successfully the duct, [Byrne et al., 2009]. As recently referred by Sjer et al. [2010], the ideal technique of common bile duct stones clearing should be minimally invasive, easy to perform, reliably clear all stones from the CBD, obtaining as well the earliest possible discharge from the hospital and leaving the patient with an undisturbed function of the papilla Vateri. The routine adoption of laparoscopic common bile duct exploration (LCBDE) associated with cholecystectomy has been promoted by the constant improvement in techniques and expertise of surgeons who are increasingly confident with laparoscopic hepato-biliary surgery and are deeply interested to bring back the whole procedure within the surgical approach. This approach seems to fulfill almost all the previous issues, nevertheless some negative aspects should be considered as the evidence that laparoscopic common bile duct surgery is time consuming and requires a rather long lasting learning curve of the whole staff of an advanced laparoscopic procedure, as well as fluoroscopic equipment and expensive accessories for the procedure that moreover may not be feasible in cases where the CBD diameter is <6 mm., [Fitzgibbons & Gardner, 2001]. Our group, as other centers, adopted the procedure of single-stage laparoscopic cholecystectomy (LC) plus common bile duct exploration, with stone extraction performed by different techniques, and a randomized prospective study has been designed to compare it with the standard double-stage procedure based on preoperative endoscopic clearance followed by a laparoscopic cholecystectomy, with the aim of assessing the more safe and successful therapy for the patient.

2. Materials and methods

In our unit from January 1996 until June 2010, 918 consecutive patients underwent elective or acute laparoscopic cholecystectomy, and ductal biliary stones were detected in 121 patients (13.1%). These patients were treated with the two-stage procedure until 2002, at that time laparoscopic common bile duct exploration and treatment, if necessary, was introduced following a decision analysis performed with the aim of evaluating cost/benefits, efficacy, recurrence, compliance of the patients as referred in the literature, [Urbach et al., 2001].
Consequently 124 out of 534 consecutive patients with evidence (36 patients) or suspicion (88 patients) of duct stones as result of a diagnostic program including US scanning , MR cholangiography and biochemical investigations, were randomly assigned to one of the two selected procedures: one-stage surgical procedure (group 1) and two-stages endoscopic + surgical procedure (group 2). All patients were informed about each procedure and involved technology and they were also asked for their consent to be randomized in the group 1 or in the group 2 and signed the consent forms. Exclusion criteria against laparoscopic common bile duct exploration were suspicion of malignancy, stone impaction, evidence of severe pancreatitis and/or cholangitis or unfitness for general anesthesia, consequently from this series were excluded three patients.
The two groups had comparable demographic and clinical profiles, (tab. 1). The presence of stones was confirmed in 39 out of 62 pts. of the two-stage group who underwent preoperative ERCP and sphincterotomy for clearing the CBD and after 2-5 days underwent a successful laparoscopic cholecystectomy. In the one–stage group stones were found in 45/62 pts. in whom an intraoperative ductal exploration was attempted via the cystic duct that was successful in 55 patients, (88.7%) and required a choledochotomy in 7 patients (11.3%), because of the size of the stones or unexpected intraoperative difficulties.
Stones were completely removed through the cystic duct in 29 patients while in 16 patients through the previous or a newly performed choledochotomy, using Dormia and/or Fogarty catheters. The transcystic approach failed because of the following reasons: the cystic duct was too small or frale, the stones were larger than 1 cm or in a number greater than five or proximal to the confluence into the hepatic duct. The techniques of transcystic catheter

insertion to extract the stones include cystic duct dilation, washing, exploration with biliary balloon catheters or wire baskets, final check with a cholangiography at the end of the procedure. In case of choledocotomy a biliary endoscopy was also performed in 9/16 patients, with an Olympus flexible choledocoscope CHF-CB 30S, in order to remove stones with a catheters under direct vision or to check the duct after the removal of the stones. All patients underwent a control cholangiogram to ensure that duct's clearance was successfully done and that the papilla was patent to contrast dye passage into the duodenum. External biliary drainage with T tube and postoperative cholangiography was performed in 9 patients. All patient had an external transparietal subhepatic drainage at least for 24 hours, at most for four-five days in those patients in which T-tube drainage was inserted, to control potential early or late persistent biliary leak. T tube was removed after a negative control with a transKehr cholangiography performed within 3-4 weeks from the previous surgery. The laparoscopic procedure was completed in 121 patients (97.6%). Patients were followed up for 1-9 years (mean 4.5 yrs.), visiting them in the outpatient clinic or interviewing by telephone calls after the first year.

2.1 Operative procedure

The laparoscopic cholecystectomy was performed with a standard four-trocar technique using the transumbilical open approach according to the Hasson technique. In case of preoperative evidence or suspicion of CBD stones, a small quantity of diluted contrast solution was injected, (Ultravist-300, Schering A.G., Berlin, Germany, 50% diluted with a 0.9% saline solution), performing the first cholangiography through the incision of the cystic duct made close to the confluence into the common duct to facilitate the passage of the operative cholangiogram catheter 4.5 Fr x 45.7cm (TAUT inc. Geneva, Il 60134 USA).

Preoperative clinical variables	LCBDE (n = 62)	ERCP +LC (n = 62)	p Value
Age (years)	53 ± 13	55 ± 15	NS
Gender (females, %)	76	79	NS
ASA	2 ± 1	2 ± 1	NS
Biliary symptoms (%)	75	70	0.01
Cholecystitis (%)	14.8	18.1	0.05
Jaundice (%)	6	20	0.01
Pancreatitis (%)	6.4	4.8	NS
Cholangitis (%)	0	1.6	0.05
Previous abdominal surgery (%)	29	32	NS

Table 1. Comparison of clinical demographics of patients in LCBD exploration and treatment group and in ERCP and LC group.

When CBD stones were detected a non-Radiopaque Karlan Balloon Catheter: 4 Fr. 2-Lumen, 60 cm, (Arrow percutaneous laparoscopic cholangiography set CS-01701; Arrow International Europe) was introduced on the anterior axillary line under the right costal margin to allow an appropriate access to the cystic duct, to remove the stones, using a flexible wire guide, if necessary, through the curved guide catheter. The choledochotomy was done after a good exposure of the liver hilus pulling up and to the right the gallbladder and lifting up the round ligament, exposing the anterior wall of the duct making a longitudinal   incision sometime helped by two 4/0 prolene stitches   lifting up the supraduodenal choledocus. The primary closure of the incision was done mainly with a running 4/0 prolene suture. Details of the surgical procedure (exploration, stones extraction, radiological and endoscopic control etc.), timing of the two-stage procedure, results and complications of surgical and endoscopic treatment were recorded.

2.2 Statistical analyses

The procedures performed in the two groups were recorded as success or failure according to the complete clearance of the CBD as showed by the final intraoperative cholangiography. The outcome of the procedures was evaluated as well, looking at different parameters: common bile duct diameter, number of stones, stone size, presence of intrahepatic stones, mean operating time, length of hospital stay. Some of these where splitted in two categories: the limit of 6 mm. was identified for the bile duct diameter, the size of 5 mm. for the stones, and the number of three for the stones. In significance testing Fischer's exact test was used for dichotomized discrete variables and the nonparametric Wilcoxon method for comparisons between means, [Stromberg et al., 2008].

2.3 Definition of success

It has been defined as primary outcome measure the successful removal of gallbladder and common bile duct clearance performing the procedures of treatment, and as secondary outcome the results in terms of specific and generic complications such as bleeding, cholangitis, bile leak or fistula, surgical-site infection, late recurrency and other medical complications.

3. Results

Removal of the stones in the two groups was successfully done in 79 patients (94%), mortality directly related to the procedures was nil (1 cardiac failure at 6 months) nor occurred major intra-operative complications in either group. In two patients, a conversion into laparotomy was necessary for intraoperative haemorrhage caused in the first by an accessory cystic artery and by a severe haemobilia in the second one. The average diameter of the common bile duct was 10.7 mm (range 6-22 mm). The mean number of stones was 3. 4 (1-10). The mean operating time in the group 1 was 160 m' (range 100-280 m'), the operation lasted significantly more time in the unsuccessful procedures and in patients undergone choledocal exploration, either as first choice or in case of failure of the transcystic approach.

Obviously patients who underwent laparoscopic common bile duct exploration had a longer operating time compared with the group undergone laparoscopic cholecystectomy alone (mean time 70 m'). T tubes were applied to patients with multiple stones (>5) and CBD diameter greater than 6 mm., at risk for retained sludge, previous attacks of cholangitis or pancreatitis, poor tissue quality secondary to duct's infection. It was removed within 3-4 weeks after a trans-Kehr cholangiography without complications neither difference in comparison with primary suture of the choledocal incision, (tab. 2).

Residual CBD stones were detected in the two groups at different intervals of time, following a routine control by an abdominal ultrasonography or magnetic resonance cholangiography. In two patients of the group 1 the stones were removed successfully by

ERC and endoscopic sphincterotomy after 6 and 8 months from previous surgery, in one patient a new laparoscopic approach (LCBDE) was performed after 30 months because suffering from symptoms referred to recurrent stones. The residual stones in the two patients of the group 2 were successfully removed by a new endoscopic approach and sphincterotomy (EST), without any local and systemic complication.

	N°	Successful (%)	Failure (%)	P value
Total number of patients	84	79 (94)	5 (6)	
CBD diameter				n.s.
≤ 6mm	31	29 (93.5)	2 (6.5)	
> 6mm	53	50 (94)	3 (6)	
Mean number of stones	3.4	2.9	5.2	0.0053*
Number of stones				<0.001^
≤3	58	57 (98)	1 (2)	
>3	26	22 (85)	4 (15)	
Mean stone size (mm)	5.4	5.1	8.3	0.0045*
Stone size				<0.001^
≤5mm	61	60 (98)	1 (2)	
>5 mm	23	19 (83)	4 (17)	
Intrahepatic stones				n.s.
Yes	3	3 (100)	0	
No	81	76 (94)	5 (6)	
Mean operating time (minutes)	170m'	150m'	230m'	<0.001^
Mean length of hospital stay (2-16days)	7.1	4.5	9.0	<0.001^

* Fischer's exact test
^Wilcoxon nonparametric method

Table 2. Overall results of the procedures of CBD stones removal

There was a significant increasing risk among patients with stones of diameter greater than 5 mm. compared to patients with stones of 5 mm. or less. One-stage management of duct stones was associated with a significant less morbidity than two-stage approach (8.1% vs. 14.2%), which is increasingly significant for multiple stones or stones > 5mm. Haemorrhage occurred in 4.8% (2.2% vs. 7.7%), pancreatitis in 2.4% (2.2% vs. 2.6), port site infection and cholangitis in 1.1% (in the group 2). The mean postoperative hospital stay was 7.1 days (range 2-16), and depended mainly on the surgical outcome in terms of clearing of the common bile duct i.e. success or failure of the procedure.

In the group 1, one patient, who underwent a transcystic stone extraction had a biliary leak not requiring reoperation. After 13 months one patient of the group 2 underwent a new endoscopic treatment, as she was referred to our Day Surgery Unit for a symptomatic cholangitis with evidence of biliary sludge by ultrasonographic examination at the casualty department, caused by a stenosis of the papilla Vateri as showed by a following magnetic resonance, (tab. 3).

	LCBDE (n=45)	ERCP +LC (n=39)	p Value
	N° (%)	N° (%)	
Successful	42 (93)	37 (95)	n.s.
Failure	3 (7)	2 (5)	
CBD diameter			n.s.
≤6mm	15 (33)	16 (41)	
>6mm	30 (67)	23 (59)	
Mean number of stones	3.5	3.2	n.s
≤3	32 (71)	26 (67)	
>3	13 (29)	13 (33)	
Mean stone size (mm)	5.2	5.7	n.s.
Stone size			
≤5mm	32 (71)	29 (74)	
>5mm	13 (29)	10 (26)	
Intrahepatic stones			
Yes	2	1	n.s.
No	43	38	
Postoperative complications	4 (8.8)	6 (15.3)	0.0045*
stone size ≤5mm	1 (2.2)	2 (5.1)	<0.005^
>5 mm	3 (6.6)	4 (10.2)	
Number ≤3	0	1	
>3	4	5	
Mean length of hospital stay (2-16days)	7.1	3.5	<0.001^

* Fischer's exact test
^Wilcoxon nonparametric method.

Table 3. Comparison of the results of stones removal between the two groups

4. Discussion

The aim of this study was to evaluate the results of the treatment of common bile duct stones in patients undergoing single-stage laparoscopic management of gallstones and CBD stones performing either transcystic common bile duct exploration (TC-CBDE) or laparoscopic choledochotomy, compared to the two-stage well established and more widely used endoscopic retrograde cholangioscopy + endoscopic sphincterotomy followed by laparoscopic cholecystectomy. The analysis of the results of this prospective study, based on a randomized distribution of 124 consecutive patients in which suspicion or evidence of CBD stones was reported, emphasizes the role of mininvasive treatment of gallbladder and CBD stones, that has become the main focus of biliary surgery. Though a single center study, a comparison has been done between two procedures, with the removal of stones from CBD as primary end-point, recruiting consecutive patients affected by common bile duct stones or highly suspected of stones presence, without any selection criteria, except the exclusion caused by malignant lesions, high surgical risks or patient's refusal to undergo surgery. They were randomly assigned either to a totally laparoscopic approach including cholecystectomy and duct exploration and treatment, if necessary, or to a double procedure: endoscopic (ERC ± EST) as first step, followed by laparoscopic cholecystectomy at different interval of time depending mainly on the outcome of the endoscopic treatment.

These are scheduled among the accepted procedures for an elective treatment, since the conservative or wait and see strategy have been ruled out. Other procedures as the association of the laparoscopic cholecystectomy with ERC + endoscopic sphincterotomy known as the rendezvous approach [Morino et al., 2006; Tricarico et al., 2002;], or the endoscopic treatment after a positive intra-operative cholangiography need more experience and good cooperation between different teams, particularly in the second issue [Hong et al., 2006], and could increase the risk of postoperative complications in both cases, included the need of a second operation if the endoscopic sphincterotomy (EST) fails, [Patel et al., 2003].Laparoscopic common bile duct exploration as single approach, requires a longer learning curve mainly because of the possibility that the procedure could become more demanding if a laparoscopic suture should be performed when the removal of stones is done via a choledocal incision, with or without T-tube placement. The other single stage procedure is the laparoendoscopic rendezvous associating laparoscopic cholecystectomy with intraoperative endoscopic retrograde cholangiography with stone extraction as a one-time therapy for gallstones and CBD stones, that according to Morino et al., (2006) had a higher success rate (95.6% v. 80%), shorter hospital stay (4.3 days v. 8 days) and lesser cost (€ 2829 v. € 3834), compared with the two stage procedure. It was recently referred that the rendezvous technique can warrant a successful treatment even in cases complicated by cholangitis or pancreatitis, with the help of a guidewire introduced through the cystic duct into the papilla that may reduce the complications secondary to the endoscopic cannulation. With this device is possible to reduce the failure rate of the retrograde cholangiography as well as the incidence of the major complication, i.e. acute pancreatitis, of the laparoendoscopic rendezvous technique compared with the sequential ERCP and LC (5% vs. 20%), as referred by El Geidie et al., (2011) who had worse results (no significant difference in failure rate) probably due the non use of the guidewire. Nevertheless with this approach it is impossible to avoid the potential complications linked to the endoscopic sphincterotomy, [Borzellino et al.,2010]. As reported before the major limits lie on the management of endoscopy together with surgery in the operating theatre, and these problems have discouraged the diffusion of this combined approach throughout surgeons interested to this disease, [Meyer et al., 1999]. It should be outlined that the rendezvous procedure should be adopted only in patients with a positive evidence of common bile duct stones, and the ideal would be to predict CBD stones without invasive tests in order to avoid unnecessary and sometime risky procedures, as today magnetic resonance cholangiography actually can obtain. It is likewise necessary to refer that skilled surgeons are able to achieve an overall satisfying outcome, performing the rendez vous procedure, which is quite overlapping with those of the one stage total laparoscopic approach, also from the point of view of the residual stones' rate, [Tranter & Thompson, 2002].

On the other hand in the literature the A.A. generally agree that the first endoscopic step of the two stage procedure is associated with a high complication rate of about 10%, mainly acute pancreatitis (3%) and a mortality rate of 4%, which could increase respectively to a maximum of 16% and 6%, by the addition of the potential complications following the surgical step, [Hong et al., 2006]. This difference could be partially explained by the length of the interval between the two procedures, which is not well defined, as even in the multicenter trial by the European Association for Endoscopic Surgery (EAES) the interval between endoscopic papillosphincterotomy and laparoscopic cholecystectomy was not specified, [Cuschieri et al.,1999]. It is referred that patients awaiting for laparocopic cholecystectomy risk a high rate of readmissions and complications due to acute cholecystitis, pancreatitis, empyema and cholangitis; de Vries et al., [2005], showed that in

Laparoscopic One-Stage vs Endoscopic Plus Laparoscopic Management of Common Bile Duct Stones –
A Prospective Randomized Study

43

case of delayed cholecystectomy, done more than two weeks after endoscopic sphincterotomy, there is a higher conversion rate, increasing from 4% when LC was done within 2 weeks, to 31% between 2 and 6 weeks, and 16% after 6 weeks. A consequence of these considerations was the policy of leaving in situ the gallstones, avoiding the second laparoscopic approach, a sort of wait and see strategy based on the results of retrospective studies which described a relatively low incidence (5–12%) of biliary complications or recurrent symptoms in patients not undergone routine cholecystectomy following the endoscopic removal of common bile duct stones, [Byrne et al., 2009]. Nevertheless there is a positive consensus on the indication to primary endoscopic sphincterotomy in case of suppurative cholangitis, severe pancreatitis, high-risk patients, and patients who had previous cholecystectomy, [NIH Consensus Statements, 2002]. In our study patients with gallstones did not undergo any invasive diagnostic exploration if not in case of history of jaundice, gallstone pancreatitis with elevated amylase or lipase, elevated bilirubin level, abnormal liver function test results, dilated CBD on preoperative ultrasonography. Magnetic resonance cholangiography was performed when were present one or more criteria above referred, which as well indicated the necessity to perform an intraoperative cholangiography (IOC). The presence of stones was confirmed in 84 out of 124 patients (68%) who entered in the prospective trial and subsequently were explored by IOC or ERCP, the rate of stones was similar in the two groups without significant difference between groups, (72% vs. 60%: p< 0.05), confirming that they were substantially homogeneous. The overall evaluation of the outcome of the two procedures shows that two factors mainly influence the results of the treatment: the number and the size of stones, neither CBD diameter neither intrahepatic stones influenced the outcome of the procedures. Strömberg et al., [2008] confirmed previous results of Petelin, [2003], who referred that patients with stones larger than 5 mm had a significant threefold increased risk of failure in stone clearance compared to patients with stones ≤ 5 mm., and suggested a causal relation between large stone size and an increased risk of failure in stone clearance during LTCE. As consequence of the difficulties come across the procedures, postoperative complications were significantly higher in patients unsuccessfully treated. Nevertheless in the overall series postoperative morbidity was reasonably low and there was no postoperative mortality among the patients enrolled in this study. All these data agree with most of the past and recent reports in the literature [Campbell et al., 2004; Kharbutli & Velanovich, 2008], confirming the indications of the European Association for Endoscopic Surgery for TC-CBDE that are limited to stones that are smaller than the size of the cystic duct [Paganini et al., 2007]. However in our experience the dilation of the cystic duct with a balloon catheter, as usually done to easy the passage into the choledochus, allows to carry out successfully the transcystic procedure for extracting stones even larger than cystic duct, moreover becase of their friability. Nevertheless the choledocothomy, performed by elective choice or compelled by intraoperative complication or difficult removal, did not imply an increase of risks and the rate of successful extraction of stones in the two groups is quite similar, without any difference statistically significant (93% vs. 95%). The learning curve of laparoscopic duct exploration (LCBDE) through choledocothomy is not negligible, but once achieved a sufficient expertise it can be safely performed during the one-stage procedure without any evidence for longer hospitalization caused directly by the surgical maneuvers on common duct. No biliary peritonitis or postoperative cholangitis were observed in the one stage group and some minor complications (hyperamylasemia, port site infection, biliary leak etc.) were treated by a conservative therapy and did not require surgical measures, as well as they did not lengthen significantly the mean hospital stay, as also showed   by the results of different authors, who did not report significant increase of common duct lesions by surgical and/or instrumental maneuvers [Decker et al., 2003; Lezoche & Paganini, 1995; Paganini et al.,   2007] . However the transcystic cannulation of the common bile duct must be regarded as the primary approach to explore CBD, and it can be done as showed by our experience in agreement with several authors, because it is less invasive than laparoscopic choledochotomy.

Nevertheless when stones are larger than 6 mm. or located above the cystic duct choledocothomy could be indicated or sometime compelled by the failure of the transcystic exploration and/or stones removal. The extraction of the stones can be very difficult when they are impacted but in most cases gentle maneuvers with atraumatic Croce forceps through the choledochotomy or irrigation with saline solutions can achieve, after some efforts, a successful duct clearing. However in case of failure biliary Fogarthy catheters or Dormia basket could be used blindly or under vision introducing a choledocoscope, through the cystic duct or more easily through the choledochotomy, depending, of course from the diameter of the endoscope available. It was referred that the mean rate of failure because of residual stones after laparoscopic exploration and treatment of duct stones is about 5%-7% , that is quite similar to the rate referred by Moreaux, [1995], following open biliary surgery. The use of choledochoscopy can reduce to 2.8% the rate of residual stones according to the experience of Berthou et al., [2007], which is remarkably lower than the incidence ranging from 17% to 35% of residual stones following endoscopic treatment [Lenriot et al., 1993; Tranter & Thompson,2002]. Recently it has been confirmed that employing the Dormia laparoscopic basket under control of a choledochoscope the CBD removal is safer and more effective as far as postoperative complication and residual stones are concerned, particularly in comparison with endoscopic procedure burdened by a 10% rate of residual stones, which is significantly higher and advised to perform non surgical treatment only in case of high risk patients, [Campagnacci et al., 2010], . There is no doubt that the direct approach to CBD can eliminate any problem caused by high number or large diameter of the stones, or their intrahepatic placement. In our experience about 35% of stones extraction was accomplished performing a choledochotomy, sutured at the end of the procedure mainly with a primary running suture. A closure over a T tube with an external biliary drainage and postoperative cholangiography was done in 9 patients, without differences in postoperative complication rate, except the necessity of a   cholangiographyc control following surgery, to check the duct's patency with normal flow of the contrast into the duodenum, and even the potential presence of residual stones, sludge or fragments of stones, which were flushed down through the papilla with saline injection, provided that there was no leak around the catheter. The procedure was repeated   before the removal of the T tube, which did not cause any major problem, such as peritonitis or biliary fistula, nor minor local or general complication.

In our experience the use of endobiliary T tube did not affect the outcome in terms of complications, even if we realize that the number of our patients is relatively poor and does not allow any definite conclusion. However in the literature it is referred that the most frequent early complications after LCBDE derive from biliary leaks or infections and are caused mainly by the presence of biliary drainage, that could also cause late biliary stricture, [Decker et al., 2003; Thompson & Tranter,2002; Alhamdani et al., 2008]. Thompson and Tranter [2002] reported a complication rate of 16% following the use of the T tube vs. 5% for primary closure. However our results support those of Paganini and Lezoche , [1998] and

Laparoscopic One-Stage vs Endoscopic Plus Laparoscopic Management of Common Bile Duct Stones –
A Prospective Randomized Study

45

Berthou et al., [2007], who found a similar incidence of biliary complications following both the procedures. It is generally accepted that a closure over a T tube is to prefer when the CBD is inflamed because of recurrent cholangitis, [Karaliotas et al., 2008], or dilated and consequently at risk of postoperative atonia and leakage, it could likewise allow for postoperative radiographic control and in case even for extraction of missed or retained stones. There are also some studies comparing primary closure versus T tube drainage which refer similar rates of complications, but definitely it was showed a shorter operating times and a consistent trend toward shorter hospital stays in favour of the primary closure, [Kanamaru et al., 2007; Jameel et al., 2008].

The incidence of residual or recurrent biliary stones, which has been referred as failure of the procedures in table 1, is quite similar in the two groups (7% vs. 5%), with a rate of residual stones sensibly lower in the LCBDE group (4.1%). These data are slightly higher than those referred by Chander et al., with a rate of 2.7%, [2011], and by Berthou et al.,[2007], of 2.8%, Paganini et al., [2007], of 3.1%, Hong et al., [2006], of 3.5%, but are lower than the rate of 6.3% of Schreurs et al., [36], and all the same are significantly lower than the data referred in the literature of the CBD stones recurrent rate of 9%-12% found at IOC after previous ERCP+EST and LC, [Pierce et al., 2008; Campagnacci et al., 2010].

Nowadays the patients suffering from gallstones with CBD stones scheduled to undergo laparoscopic cholecystectomy may be treated by peri-operative ERCP or managed by LCBDE associated with cholecystectomy in a single surgical step. The "Guidelines on the management of common bile duct stones (CBDS)" [Williams et al., 2008], asserted that "There is no evidence of a difference in efficacy, morbidity or mortality when these approaches are compared, though LCBDE is associated with a shorter hospital stay. It is recommended that the two approaches are considered equally valid treatment options, and that training of surgeons in LCBDE is to be encouraged. (Evidence grade I b. Recommendation grade A.)". It seems that it is widely accepted the evidence from randomised control trials that the outcomes of the one- and two-stage procedures are comparable, some arguments in favour of laparoscopic exploration of the biliary duct could be the evidence of a shorter hospital stay and a better cost-effectiveness as showed by Urbach et al., [2001]. However data from the Cochrane Hepato-Biliary Group, [Martin et al., 2006], don't support any definite evidence of superiority in terms of efficacy, morbidity and mortality of one procedure over another, while the metanalysis of the literature had showed clearly that open biliary surgery was significantly superior to ERC+Endoscopic sphincterotomy in achieving CBD stone clearance.

Recently the Practice/Clinical Guidelines published on 01/2010 by the Society of American Gastrointestinal and Endoscopic Surgeons: "SAGES guidelines for the clinical application of laparoscopic biliary tract surgery" in the chapter dedicated to the management of choledocholithiasis stated that:

- There are several approaches and current data does not suggest clear superiority of any one approach. (Level I, Grade A).
- Laparoscopic transcystic common bile duct exploration is frequently successful, but may be hampered by analomous anatomy, proximal stones, strictures and large or numerous stones. (Level II, Grade B).
- Laparoscopic choledochotomy requires advanced laparoscopic skills, but has good clearance rates; the incision may be closed over a T tube, an exteriorized transcystic drain, or primary closure with or without endoluminal drainage. (Level II, Grade B).

- ERCP with stone extraction may be performed selectively before, during or after cholecystectomy with little discernable difference in morbidity and mortality and similar clearance rates when compared to laparoscopic common bile duct exploration, though routinely performed preoperative ERCP will likely result in unnecessary procedures with higher than acceptable mortality and morbidity rates. (Level I, Grade A).

On the basis of this evidence based medicine, our experience from the results of this trial suggests that biliary stones should be treated again by surgeons in first approach, as the endoscopic procedures do not automatically guarantee the complete cleansing of choledocus from stones or the absence of endoscopically related complications. Consequently a surgeon used to perform laparoscopic advanced procedures and dedicated to the management of hepato-biliary diseases, should improve his skill in the intraoperative management of the common bile duct, because the treatment of the individual patient needs an available and expert surgical team to assure good results in terms of success, costs, and length of hospital stay.

The experience resulting from this prospective study supports the aim of demonstrating that laparoscopic surgery of cholecystocholedocal stones is as safe as the procedure associating LC with endoscopic removal of ductstones, but in the great majority of cases it avoids an unnecessary double admission to the hospital services, lowers the risks connected with a double procedure, and as far as the outcome of the follow-up, though not too extended, it involves a low recurrence rate, as already showed in a study with a long-term follow-up (118 mo.) by Paganini et al., [2007]. Looking at the clinical effectiveness, and at the cost/benefits ratio, these two procedures should be considered therefore between the most useful treatment of biliary stones disease, but the single surgical approach has the advantage of taking care of the papilla Vateri avoiding unnecessary and sometimes dangerous sphincterotomy, [Sugiyama & Atomi, 2002].

Differently from the observation referred by Hong et al., [2006], about the use of the cholangioscope to remove the stones, because it could cause a waste of time, we would stress the opinion that all the techniques and devices used in the open approach to common bile duct, which are currently available in the up-to-date models, should be as well at disposal of the laparoscopic exploration of the bile duct, and used by the surgeon depending on the needs more than on predisposed patterns. The ability of managing even difficult situations consists in choosing the better way to explore the duct and to remove the stones if identified, without rejecting any helpful option. Actually most of the authors agree on the necessity of an adequate training of the surgeon facing with laparoscopic exploration of common duct in order to allow that this procedure could become the first choice approach to biliary stones disease, preventing the occurrence of early and late complications. Our study reaches a collateral not prevented aim, demonstrating that it is possible to obtain a successful surgical treatment adopting the transcystic exploration as first-line approach, that was successful in managing common bile duct stones in almost 70% of cases and that opening the common duct in case of difficulties or failure actually increases the overall success rate of the surgical approach. This confirms the conclusion of the study of Hanif et al., [2010], who encouraged surgeons to learn and apply both the procedures when they perform the one stage laparoscopic common bile duct exploration.

5. Conclusions

The significant and progressive improvements during the last decade of the diagnostic equipments associated with a definite trend to limit, as far as possible, any invasive

Laparoscopic One-Stage vs Endoscopic Plus Laparoscopic Management of Common Bile Duct Stones –
A Prospective Randomized Study

47

instrumental exploration in favour of the digital work out of the images registered by ultrasonography and magnetic resonance, has shown that it is possible to achieve excellent diagnostic results which allow a correct therapeutic approach. In a similar way the applications of new technologic devices, mainly dedicated to laparoscopic surgery, in association with the increasing diffusion of intraoperative surgical maneuvers borrowed from open surgery such as cholangiography, X-guided explorations, US scanning and others, allow the surgeons to increase their confidence with advanced laparoscopic surgery, while keeping the concepts related to a miniinvasive attitude. This study demonstrates that it is possible to deal with gallstones and CBD stones at the same time, treating them with only one surgical procedure, avoiding unnecessary damage to the papilla Vateri as well as the risk of increasing complications caused by the potential addition of the complications of the endoscopic sphincterotomy to the laparoscopic cholecystectomy, (sphincterotomy, incidentally, was a matter of violent discussions between surgeons in the past decades), and achieving a complete clearing of the common bile ducts with a low rate of residual or recurrent stones. In our study CBD clearing was done in some cases with the help of the choledocoscope, which is a safe but not crucial procedure, provided that several tricks can be used to achieve the same results, from gentle papillary pneumatic dilatation, to flush saline irrigations in association with intraductal lidocaine or intravenous glucagon administration. The peculiar friability of bile stones in the majority of cases helps the happy outcome of the whole procedure, which can be done for the most part by the transcystic route, as clearly showed by our results. Particularly the comparison between the totally surgical and the mixed endoscopic plus surgical treatment in this study did not showed a definite statistical advantage of one over the other, but it demonstrates that the one stage laparoscopic approach is able to solve the problem without mortality, with a low rate of morbidity and long distance sequences, residual stones included and finally with an earlier recovery and return to the normal activity of the patient. It is useful to outline that the one stage surgery does not complain of any of the peculiar biliary complication as cholangitis , papillary stenosis or recurrent pancreatitis referred to the endoscopic sphincterotomy, as the results our follow-up show. However we agree with the opinion that the two procedures are not in conflict each other, because it is possible to distinguish different indications, namely the general conditions of the patients, which could contraindicate a longer surgical approach, such as the laparoscopic exploration and cleaning of the common bile duct, particularly in case of previously recognized necessity of performing a choledocotomy because of size, number, position of the stones, or the local acute complications like cholangitis or stone impaction, with whom endoscopic treatment with sphincterotomy and or naso-biliary drainage more easily can deal successfully. In conclusion nowadays LCBDE is a safe and effective procedure that can be regarded as the first option approach to the treatment of patients affected by gallstones in association with CBD stones, in the hands of well experienced miniinvasive surgeons.

Disclosures: Prof. Giuseppe P. Ferulano, Drs. Saverio Dilillo, Michele D'Ambra, Ruggero Lionetti, Piero Di Silverio, Stefano Capasso, Domenico Pelaggi, Michele Rutigliano, have no conflicts of interest or financial ties to disclose.

6. References

Alhamdani A, Mahmud S, Jameel M, Baker A. Primary closure of choledochotomy after emergency laparoscopic common bile duct exploration. Surg Endosc 2008; 22: 2190-5.

Attili AF, De Santis A, Capri R, Repice AM, Maselli S. The natural history of gallstones: the experience. The GREPCO Group. Hepatology 1995;21:655–60.

Barbara L, Sama C, Morselli-Labate AM, Taroni F, Rusticali AG. A population study on the prevalence of gallstone disease: the Sirmione study. Hepatology 1987;7:913-917.

Bateson MC. Gallstones and cholecystectomy in modern Britain. Postgrad Med J 2000;76:700-3.

Berthou J C, Dron B, Charbonneau P, Moussalier K, Pellissier L. Evaluation of laparoscopic treatment of common bile duct stones in a prospective series of 505 patients: indications and results. Surg Endosc 2007; 21:1970–1974.

Borzellino G, Rodella L, Saladino E, Catalano F, Politi L, Minicozzi A, Cordiano C. Treatment for retrieved common bile duct stones during laparoscopic cholecystectomy: the rendezvous technique. Arch Surg. 2010; 145(12):1145-9.

Byrne MF, McLoughlin MT, Mitchell RM, Gerke H, Pappas TN, Branch MS, Jowell P S, Baillie J. The fate of patients who undergo "preoperative" ERCP to clear known or suspected bile duct stones. Surg Endosc 2009; 23:74–79.

Campagnacci R, Baldoni A, Baldarelli M, Rimini M, De Sanctis A, Di Emiddio M, Guerrieri M. Is laparoscopic fiberoptic choledochoscopy for common bile duct stones, a fine option or a mandatory step? Surg Endosc 2010; 24:547–553.

Campbell S, Mee A, Thompson MH. Common bile duct calculi-ERCP versus laparoscopic exploration. Ann R Coll Surg Engl 2004; 86:470–473.

Chander J, Vindal A, Lal P, Gupta N, Kumar Ramteke V. Laparoscopic management of CBD stones: an Indian experience. Surg Endosc 2011; 25:172–181.

Clayton ESJ, Connor S, Alexakis N, Leandros E. Meta-analysis of endoscopy and surgery versus surgery alone for common bile duct stones with the gallbladder in situ. Br J Surg 2006;93:1185–91.

Cuschieri A, Lezoche E, Morino M, Croce E, Lacy A, Toouli J, Faggioni A, Ribeiro VM, Jakimowicz J, Visa J, Hanna GB. E.A.E.S. multicenter prospective randomized trial comparing two-stage vs single-stage management of patients with gallstone disease and ductal calculi. Surg Endosc 1999; 13:952-957.

Decker G, Borie F, Millat B, Berthou JC, Deleuze A, Drouard F, Guillon F, Rodier JG, Fingerhut A. One hundred laparoscopic choledochotomies with primary closure of the common bile duct. Surg Endosc 2003; 17: 12–18.

de Vries A, Donkervoor SC, van Geloven AAW, Pierik EGJM. Conversion rate of laparoscopic cholecystectomy after endoscopic retrograde cholangiography in the treatment of choledocholithiasis. Does the time interval matter? Surg Endosc 2005; 19:996–1001.

ElGeidie AA, ElEbidy GK, Naeem YM. Preoperative versus intraoperative endoscopic sphincterotomy for management of common bile duct stones. Surg Endosc 2011; 25:1230-1237.

Everhart JE, Khare M, Hill M, Maurer KR., Prevalence and ethnic differences in gallbladder disease in the United States. Gastroenterology 1999;117:632-9.

Fitzgibbons RJ Jr, Gardner GC Laparoscopic surgery and the common bile duct. World J Surg 2001; 25:1317-132.

Jameel M, Darmas B, Baker AL. Trend towards primary closure following laparoscopic exploration of the common bile duct. Ann R Coll Surg Engl 2008; 90:29-35.

Kanamaru T, Sakata K, Nakamura Y, Yamamoto M, Ueno N, Takeyama Y. Laparoscopic choledochotomy in management of choledocholithiasis. Surg Laparosc Endosc Percutan Tech 2007;17:262-6.

Karaliotas C, Sgourakis G, Goumas C, Papaioannou N, Lilis C, Leandros E. Laparoscopic common bile duct exploration after failed endoscopic stone extraction. Surg Endosc 2008; 22:1826-31.

Kharbutli B, Velanovich V. Management of preoperative suspected choledocholithiasis: a decision analysis. J Gastrointest Surg 2008; 12:1973– 1980 .

Gracie WA, Ransohoff DF. The natural history of silent gallstones: the innocent gallstone is not a myth. N Engl J Med 1982;307:798–800.

Hanif F, Ahmed Z, Samie AM, Nassar AHM. Laparoscopic transcystic bile duct exploration: the treatment of first choice for common bile duct stones. Surg Endosc 2010; 24:1552–1556.

Hong DF, Xin Y, Chen DW (2006) Comparison of laparoscopic cholecystectomy combined with intraoperative endoscopic sphincterotomy and laparoscopic exploration of the common bile duct for cholecystocholedocholithiasis. Surg Endosc 20:424–427.

Lenriot JP, Le Neel JC, Hay JM, Jaeck D, Millat B, Fagniez PL. Cholangio-pancreatographie retrograde et sphincterotomie endoscopique pour lithiase biliaire. Gastroenterol Clin Biol 1993; 17:244–250.

Lezoche E, Paganini AM. Single-stage laparoscopic treatment of gallstones and common bile duct stones in 120 unselected, consecutive patients. Surg Endosc 1995; 9: 1070–1075.

Liu TH, Consorti ET, Kawashima A. Patient evaluation and management with selective use of magnetic resonance cholangiography and endoscopic retrograde cholangiopancreatography before laparoscopic cholecystectomy. Ann Surg 2001;234:33–40.

Macadam RCA, Goodall RJR Long-term symptoms following endoscopic sphincterotomy for common bile duct stones. Surg Endosc 2004; 18: 363–366

Martin DJ, Vernon DR, Toouli J. Surgical versus endoscopic treatment of bile duct stones. Cochrane Database Syst Rev 2006 (2): CD003327.

Meyer C, Vo Huu Le J, Rohr S. Management of common bile duct stones in a single operation combining laparoscopic cholecystectomy and perioperative endoscopic sphincterotomy. Surg Endosc 1999; 13:874–87.

Moreaux J. Traditional surgical management of common bile duct stones: a prospective study during a 20 year experience. Am J Surg 1995; 169: 220–226.

Morino M, Baracchi F, Miglietta C, Furlan N, Ragona R, Garbarini A. Preoperative endoscopic sphincterotomy versus laparoendoscopic rendezvous in patients with gallbladder and bile duct stones. Ann Surg 2006;244:889–96.

National Institutes of Health (NIH) state of the science on endoscopic retrograde cholangiopancreatography (ERCP) for diagnosis and therapy. NIH Consens Sci Statements 2002; 19: 1–26.

Paganini AM, Lezoche E. Follow-up of 161 unselected consecutive patients treated laparoscopically for common bile duct stones. Surg Endosc 1998; 12: 23–29.

Paganini A M, Guerrieri M, Sarnari J, De Sanctis A, D'Ambrosio G, Lezoche G, Perretta S, Lezoche E. Thirteen years experience with laparoscopic transcystic common bile duct exploration for stones. Effectiveness and long-term results. Surg Endosc (2007) 21: 34–40.

Patel AP, Lokey JS, Harris JB, Sticca RP, McGill ES, Arrillaga A, Miller RS, Kopelman TR. Current management of common bile duct stones in a teaching community hospital. Am Surg 2003;69:555–560.

Petelin JB. Laparoscopic common bile duct exploration. Surg Endosc 2003; 17: 1705–1715.

Pierce RA, Jonnalagadda S, Spitler JA, Tessier DJ, Liaw JM, Lal SC, Melman LM, Frisella MM, Todt LM, Brunt LM, Halpin VJ, Eagon JC, Edmundowicz SA, Matthews BD. Incidence of residual choledocholithiasis detected by intraoperative cholangiography at the time of laparoscopic cholecystectomy in patients having undergone preoperative ERCP. Surg Endosc 2008; 22:2365– 2372.

Pixley F, Wilson D, McPherson K, Mann J., Effect of vegetarianism on development of gall stones in women. BMJ (Clin Res Ed) 1985;291:11–2.

Schreurs WH, Juttmann JR, . Stuifbergen WNHM, Oostvogel HJM and Vroonhoven TJMV. Management of common bile duct stones . Surg Endosc 2002; 16, 1068–1072.

Sjer A. EB, Boland DM, van Rijn PJJ, Mohamad S. A decade of washing out common bile duct stones with papillar balloon dilatation as a one-stage procedure during laparoscopic cholecystectomy. Surg Endosc 2010; 24:2226–2230.

Stromberg C, Nilsson M, Leijonmarck CE. Stone clearance and risk factors for failure in laparoscopic transcystic exploration of the common bile duct. Surg Endosc 2008; 22:1194–1199.

Sugiyama M, Atomi Y. Risk factors predictive of late complications after endoscopic sphincterotomy for bile duct stones: long-term (more than 10 years) follow-up study. Am J Gastroenterol 2002; 97: 2763–2767.

Thompson MH, Tranter SE. All-comers policy for laparoscopic exploration of the common bile duct. Br J Surg 2002; 89: 1608–1612.

Tranter SE, Thompson MH Comparison of endoscopic sphincterotomy and laparoscopic exploration of the common bile duct. Br J Surg 2002; 89: 1495–1504.

Tricarico A, Cione G, Sozio M, Di Palo P, Bottino V, Tricarico T,Tartaglia A, Iazzetta I, Sessa E, Mosca S, De Nucci C, Falco P. Endolaparoscopic rendezvous treatment: a satisfying therapeutic choice for cholecystocholedocholithiasis. Surg Endosc 2002; 16: 585–588.

Urbach DR, Khajanchee YS, Jobe BA, Standage BA, Hanson PD, Swanstrom LL. Cost-effective management of common bile duct stones. A decision analysis of the use of endoscopic retrograde cholangiopancreatography (ERCP), intraoperative cholangiography and laparoscopic bile duct exploration. Surg Endosc 2001; 15:4–13.

Williams EJ, Green J, Beckingham I, Parks R, Martin D, Lombard M. Guidelines on the management of common bile duct stones (CBDS). Gut 2008;57:1004-21.

3

Endoscopic Ultrasound for Solid and Cystic Neoplasms of the Pancreas

Karim M. Eltawil[1] and Michele Molinari[2]
*[1]Dalhousie University, Department of Surgery, Queen Elizabeth II
Health Sciences Centre, Rm 6-302 Victoria Building,Halifax, Nova Scotia
[2]Associate Professor of Surgery, Rm 6-302 Victoria Building, Halifax, Nova Scotia
Canada*

1. Introduction

Endoscopic ultrasound (EUS) was introduced in clinical practice in 1980[1] and during the last few decades the quality of instrumentation has improved significantly. The first commercially available radial echoendoscope was introduced in Japan [2] and then in Europe [3] in the mid to late 1980s. At that time, radial probes were used for fine needle aspiration (FNA). Only in the early 1990s EUS-FNA become technologically practical with the introduction of linear echoendoscopes that generated ultrasonic images parallel to the shaft of the instrument. With this modification, needles could be guided into areas of interest. Soon after this improvement, the first report of EUS-FNA of the pancreas was published [4] and numerous other publications have followed [5-8]. Later on, mechanical probes have been replaced by electrical probes that allowed expansion of the diagnostic capacity of EUS. More recently, the addition of color Doppler ultrasonography, injection of contrasts for ultrasound and the application of elastography has further extended the clinical use of EUS for hepatobiliary and pancreatic diseases. The fact that EUS is able to provide direct visualization of the walls of the gastrointestinal tract and direct the placement of needles for cytology or histology specimens [5,9], makes this technique very useful for the diagnosis of benign and malignant diseases of these organs that are difficult to reach percutaneouly. In recent years diagnostic modalities such as multidetector-multiphasic CT with pancreatic protocols, magenetic resonance imaging (MRI) and positron emission tomography (PET) scans have improved significantly the pre-operative tumor staging of pancreatic malignancies. Nevertheless, a significant proportion of patients will benefit from EUS-FNA for confirmation of pancreatic neoplasm and assessment of the planes along the vascular superior mesenteric trunk[10].

2. Epidemiology of pancreatic neoplasms

Pancreatic adenocarcinoma is the fourth leading cause of cancer related mortality in the United States with estimated 42,500 new cases and 35,000 deaths from the disease each year [11]. In industrialized countries, the incidence of pancreatic adenocarcinoma (11 per 100,000 individuals) ranks second after colorectal cancer among all gastrointestinal malignances[12]. More than 80% of PCs are diagnosed in patients older than 60 and almost 50% have distant metastases at the time of presentation[13,14]. Men are more frequently affected than women

(Relative Risk (RR) = 1.3) and individuals of African American descent in comparison to Caucasians (RR= 1.5) [15]. Analysis of overall survival shows that the prognosis of PC is still quite poor despite the fact that 1-year survival has increased from 15.2% (period between 1977-1981) to 21.6% (period between 1997-2001) and 5-year survival has increased from 3% (period between 1977-1986) to 5% (period between 1996-2004)[16].

3. Classification of pancreatic neoplasms

The vast majority (90%) of pancreatic cancers (PC) are malignant tumors originating from pancreatic ductal cells [17]. Anatomically, 78% of PCs are located in the head, and the remaining 22% are equally distributed in the body and in the tail[18]. The most common

EPITHELIAL TUMORS	NON-EPITHELIAL TUMORS
Benign Pancreatic Tumors	**Endocrine Tumors**
Serous Cystoadenoma	Insulinoma (Incidence: 70-80%)
Mucinous Cystoadenoma	Gastrinoma (Incidence: 20-25%)
Intraductal Papillary Mucinous Neoplasm (IPMN)	VIPoma (Incidence: 4%)
Mature Teratoma	Glucagonoma (Incidence: 4%)
Borderline Pancreatic Tumors	Somastatinoma (Incidence: <5%)
Mucinous Cystic Neoplasm with Moderate Dysplasia	Carcinoid (Incidence: <1%)
Intraductal Papillary Mucinous Neoplasm with Moderate Dysplasia	ACTHoma (Incidence: <1%)
Solid-pseudopapillary Neoplasm (SPPN)	GRFoma (Incidence: <1%)
Malignant	PTH-like-oma (Incidence: <1%)
Ductal Adenocarcinoma	Neurotensinoma (Incidence: <1%)
Mucinous non-cystic carcinoma	Non-functional tumors (Incidence 30-50%)
Signet ring cell carcinoma	**Mesenchymal Neoplasms**
Undifferentiated (anaplastic) carcinoma	Leiomyoma
Undifferentiated carcinoma with osteoclast-like giant cells	Lipoma
Mixed ductal-endocrine carcinoma	Neurofibroma - Ganglioneuromas
Serous Cystoadenocarcinoma	Hemangyoma - Lymphangioma
Mucinous Cystoadenocarcinoma	Granular Cell Tumors
Intraductal Papillary-Mucinous Carcinoma	Schwann Cell Tumors
Acinar Cell Carcinoma	Gastrointestinal Stroma Tumors (GIST)
Medullary Carcinoma	B-cell Lymphomas
Acinar Cell Cystoadenocarcinoma	**Metastatic Tumors**
Pancreatoblastoma	Renal Cell Carcinoma
Solid-pseudopapillary Carcinoma	Melanoma
Others	Breast Cancer
	Squamous Cell Carcinoma
Secondary Tumors	Endometrioid Adenocarcinoma
	Osteosarcoma

Table 1. Tumor Classification

clinical presentations are progressive weight loss and anorexia, mid abdominal pain and jaundice. Pancreatic neoplasms are classified in benign or malignant according to the cytological characteristics. These can be further divided into endocrine or exocrine tumors according to the function of their cells and into cystic or solid according to the macroscopic features of the lesion. Recent advances in surgical pathology techniques integrated with molecular biology have allowed advances in the modern classification of pancreatic neoplasms. A summary of the clinico-pathological features of the different categories of pancreatic lesions is shown in **Table 1**.

4. Conventional diagnostic modalities for pancreatic cancer

4.1 Abdominal ultrasound
Trans-abdominal ultrasound (US) is often used as a screening test [19]. Its sensitivity ranges between 48% [8] and 89% [20] with accuracy between 46% [8] and 64%[21]. Small tumors measuring less than 1cm are detected by US in only 50% of cases while the sensitivity increases to 95.8% for tumors larger than 3 cm[20]. US has a relatively low performance profile for staging of pancreatic tumors as its sensitivity for lymph nodes involvement ranges only between 8 [17] to 57 % [20]. Color Doppler US has been used to assess possible involvement of the portal vein and superior mesenteric vessels with a sensitivity ranging between 50% [22] and 94% [23] specificity between 80% and 100% [22] and accuracy between 81% and 95% [19].

4.2 Computed Tomography
On contrast CT, pancreatic adenocarcinoma appears as an ill-defined, hypo attenuating focal mass with dilatation of the upstream pancreatic and or biliary duct [24]. The optimum visualization of the pancreas requires imaging acquisition obtained during both arterial and portal phases [25] with sensitivity and specificity of 77% and 100% respectively for lesions less than 2 cm [26]. In a multicentric trial, the diagnostic accuracy of contrast CT for resectability was 73% with 90% PPV for non resectability [27]. With the advent of multi detector CT scanners (MDCT) the pancreas can be imaged at a very high spacial and temporal resolution[28,29]. Recent studies have shown that NPV for respectability was 87% for MDCT compared to 79% for conventional helical CT [30] and with accuracy between 85% and 95% [31,32].

4.3 Magnetic Resonance Imaging (MRI-MRCP)
In most institutions, MRI is performed when other imaging modalities provide insufficient data for the clinical staging of the tumor or when treatment planning can not be based on the images obtained by other techniques. Several studies have shown that MRI is superior to CT scan for the detection and staging of pancreatic adenocarcinoma (100% vs. 94% respectively)[33-36]. The use of MRI-MRCP for pancreatic malignancies is supported by a prospective analysis showing that MRI-MRCP was superior to CT in differentiating malignant from benign lesions and MRI-MRCP had better sensitivity (92% vs. 76%), specificity (85% vs. 69%), accuracy (90% vs. 75%), PPV (95% vs. 88%) and NPV (79% vs. 50%) compared to CT [37].

4.4 Positron Emission Tomography
[18]F-2fluoro-2-deoxy-D-glucose (FDG) accumulated by tumor cells provides PET the advantage of combining metabolic activity and imaging characteristics. Newly developed PET scanners can detect small PC up to 7mm in diameter and diagnose metastatic disease in

about 40% of cases[38,39]. A Japanese study found that the overall sensitivity of PET-CT was superior to contrast CT (92% vs. 88%) and that PET was better at detecting bone metastases (100% vs. 12%). However, CT scan was superior for the evaluation of vascular invasion (100% vs. 22%), involvement of para-aortic regional lymph nodes (78% vs. 57%), identification of peritoneal dissemination (57% vs. 42%) and hepatic metastases (73% vs. 52%) [40].

4.5 Treatment of pancreatic neoplasms

Solid tumors of the pancreas are typically associated with malignancy, whereas cystic tumors more often tend to be benign[41]. Due to the difficulties in differentiating benign from malignant lesions, resection is often indicated when patient's conditions and tumor stage allows it [42]. Surgical resection with negative margins is the only potential curative treatment for pancreatic malignancies but unfortunately, even when surgery is performed successfully, recurrent disease is frequent and long term survival is expected only for 5-15% of patients[17]. According to the United States Surveillance and Epidemiology End Results registries, the 5-year relative survival for the period between 1999 and 2006 was 22.5% for localized and 1.9% for metastatic tumors [43]. The majority of tumors are diagnosed when locally advanced or with early metastases, and only 20% are suitable for resection at the time of diagnosis. Despite the improvements in surgical techniques and advances in perioperative supportive care that have reduced the mortality rates to less than 5% in high volume centers, pancreatic surgery remains challenging [44-46]. Therefore, pre-operative accurate staging is fundamental in identifying patients who would benefit from surgery. EUS has been shown to play an important role in preoperative diagnosis and tumor staging as it provides high resolution images of the pancreas without interference of bowel gas [47].

4.6 EUS equipment and techniques

EUS is usually performed with patients positioned in the left dcubitus and under conscious sedation. The transducer located in the tip of the oblique-viewing fiberscope is inserted as far as the second portion of the duodenum, and scanning is done with a de-areated water filled ballon applied to the tip of the echoendoscope. After examination of the pancreatic head, the ecoendoscope is drawn backward to the stomach, and EUS of the body and tail of the pancreas is performed. The frequency usually used to assess the pancreas and surrounding organs during EUS ranges between 5 and 12 MHz [48]. During the last decade, intraductal US (IDUS) has been possible by the introduction of miniprobes measuring 1.7-2.4 mm in outer diameter that can be advanced in the common bile and pancreatic ducts utilizing scanning frequencies ranging between 10-30MHz and obtaining a maximum tissue view penetration of approximately 2 cm [1,48]. The miniprobe is initially introduced into the papilla of Vater and advanced into the pancreatic or bile duct beyond the area of interest and then it is slowly pulled back. The location of the miniprobe can be confirmed by using fluoroscopy as it is usually done during regular endoscopic retrograde cholangio-pancreatography (ERCP). IDUS is able to visualize only limited parts of the pancreas and surrounding structure such as the splenic vessels, portal vein, superior mesenteric artery and vein and extrahepatic duct.

4.7 Indications for Endoscopic Ultrasound and Fine Needle Aspiration (EUS-FNA)

The most common indication for EUS-FNA of the pancreas is for evaluation of pancreatic masses with atypical characterisitics on cross sectional images or for optimal pre-operative staging (**Table 2**). Differential diagnosis of pancreatic masses includes malignant and benign neoplasms, chronic pancreatitis, lymphoma and metastases. Approximately 90% of pancreatic neoplasms are adenocarcinomas, 5% are cystic lesions, and 2-5% are neuroendocrine tumors. Metastatic lesions to the pancreas, primarily from renal cancer, lung cancer, and lymphomas represent a small percentage. Because cystadenocarcinomas[49] and neuroendocrine tumors[50] have a significantly better prognoses than pancreatic adenocarcinoma, accurate cytologic preoperative identification can significantly alter the subsequent management of these patients[51]. In general, EUS has been shown to be superior to CT, MRI, and ERCP [52] in the diagnosis of pancreatic diseases as an imaging modality [2,5,53,54]. The current sensitivity of EUS is in the range of 95-100%. During the last decades, the diagnostic advantages of EUS for pancreatic pathology have been challenged by the advances of other cross sectional modalities such as CT, MRI and PET scans [55] [56]. When combined with FNA capabilities, EUS has the advantage of being able to sample suspicious lesions. The one area where malignancies can be still easily missed by EUS, even with EUS-FNA, is in the setting of underlying chronic pancreatitis[4,53,57-59]. No single or combination of imaging modalities has yet proven accurate in definitively determining when a patient with chronic pancreatitis has developed pancreatic cancer. The technique of EUS-guided FNA involves passing an 18 to 22 gauge metal needle through the biopsy port of a linear echoendoscope under real-time guidance into an endosonographically visualized pancreatic mass. The needle is then moved back and forth several times (5-10 passes) with varying degrees of negative pressure to collect cells or small tissue samples that are then deposited on cytology slides for immediate fixation and staining [60]. EUS-FNA of primary pancreatic malignancies is able to provide a definitive diagnosis in 80-93% of cases [8,54,57,61-63]. The ability to have a cytopathologist on site who can provide immediate feedback on the quality and adequacy of the specimens obtained by FNA is extremely important for the accurate diagnosis[62,63]. Choosing what part of a pancreatic mass to aspirate is something of an art and comes with experience. The most difficult pancreatic masses to aspirate are the ones located near the uncinate process as it can be very hard to direct the needle to enter the lesion around the second and third portion of the duodenum. The best yield of diagnostic cells usually seems to come from 1 cm to 2 cm deep to the margin of the tumor. Color flow Doppler can be used prior to EUS-FNA to help avoid vessels overlying the proposed path of the aspiration needle such as are seen when there is underlying portal vein or splenic vein obstruction. Similarly to CT and ultrasound-guided FNA or biopsy, the overall complication rate secondary to EUS-FNA of the pancreas is about 1-2% [6,8,58,61,64]. The major complications reported with EUS-FNA are bleeding, pancreatitis, and infection but mortality is very rare

Indications for EUS
Acute onset of diabetes in elderly patients
Involuntary weight loss
Presence of epigastric or back pain
Acute or chronic pancreatitis
Suspected pancreatic cancer on other cross sectional imaging modalities
Family history of pancreatic cancer or presence of genetic predisposition to pancreatic cancer

Table 2. Common Indications for Endoscopic Ultrasound

and usually caused by uncontrollable hemorrhage[65] that is more likely when the patient has portal hypertension. Pancreatitis after EUS-FNA is most likely to occur in patients already being evaluated for recurrent pancreatitis and when the FNA needle is passed through more than 2 cm to 3 cm of normal pancreas to obtain a specimen. Bacteremia following EUS-FNA for solid tumors is quite uncommon while EUS-FNA of cystic pancreatic lesions has a higher risk of infectious complications and broad-spectrum intravenous antibiotics are routinely recommended. The risk of cancer seeding by EUS-FNA appears to be significantly lower when compared to percutaneous FNA [66].

4.8 EUS-FNA for benign pancreatic lesions
Indications and impact of EUS-FNA for benign disease other than pancreatic cystic lesions is still in evolution as it appears to be safe but does not add significantly to the diagnostic accuracy of EUS or other cross sectional imaging tests[67].

4.9 Ultrasonographic characteristics
Pancreatic adenocarcinoma often appears as a mass with irregular echogenicity due to the irregulary arranged carcinomatous canaliculi or coagulative necrosis of the neoplastic cells superimposed on a hypoechoic background [68]. Small pancreatic cancers instead, can often have homogeneous and hypoechoic echogeneicity that can mimic benign diseases such as focal pancreatitis, pseudotumors or islet cell neoplasms that have clear margins, smooth contour and regular central echogenicity[48]. When compared to CT scan and ERCP, EUS performs better for the detection of small pancreatic cancers (less than 2 cm in diameter) and it is currently indicated when patients are suspected to have early stage tumors or when undergoing screening for familial pancreatic cancer as it is the most sensitive diagnostic test for lesions measuring less than 1 cm in diameter [69,70].

5. Differential diagnosis of pancreatic lesions

Differentiation between pancreatic malignancies from inflammatory masses has been very challenging with the use of cross sectional imaging modalities such as US, CT scans, MRI and ERCP. EUS-FNA appears to be the best diagnostic strategy as it combines the ability of ultrasound imaging of the pancreatic lesions and the ability of obtaining samples for cytological or histological evaluation. Recent studies have reported that adequate specimen acquisition is possible in 97% of cases with accurate differential diagnosis in 87% of patients [48]. Sensitivity, specificity, positive predictive value and negative predictive value for EUS-FNA were: 85%,100%, 100% and 53% respectively[48] (**Table 3**). One of the major pitfalls is over interpretation of a lesion as positive for malignancy as a result of contamination of dysplastic cells when the needle traverses an area of high-grade dysplasia of the gastrointestinal tract mucosa. It is equally important that benign mucosal glandular cells in the aspirate of the lymph node not be over interpreted as metastasis. Although EUS-FNA is a very useful diagnostic technique for the differential diagnosis of patients with pancreatic lesions, it has to be kept in mind that even if the results of the test are negative for malignancy, pancreatic cancer can not be completely excluded. Currently, EUS-FNA should be still used in conjuction with other imaging modalities and repeated when clinical suspicion is suggestive for the possibility of malignancy (**Table 4**).

Diagnostic Performance	CT	EUS	EUS-FNA
Sensitivity	63-84%	95-100%	79-95%
Specificity	35-93%	19-81%	69-100%
Negative Predictive Value	12-49%	48-100%	31-78%
Positive Predictive Value	89-99%	85-98%	94-100%
Accuracy	70-88%	97-98%	81-96%

Table 3. Diagnsostic Performance of Endoscopic Ultrasound and Computerized Tomography for Solid Pancreatic Cancers

		CT	EUS	EUS-FNA
General Performance	Sensitivity	63-84%	95-100%	79-95%
	Negative Predictive Value	12-49%	48-100%	31-78%
	Positive Predictive Value	89-99%	85-98%	94-100%
	Accuracy	70-88%	97-98%	81-96%
Obstructive Jaundice	Sensitivity	51-80%	92-100%	71-94%
	Specificity	16-100%	1-99%	16-100%
	Negative Predictive Value	1-36%	25-100%	3-60%
	Positive Predictive Value	88-100%	88-100%	91-100%
	Accuracy	53-81%	89-100%	72-94%
Absence of Obstructive Jaundice	Sensitivity	70-98%	87-100%	80-100%
	Specificity	24-91%	16-84%	63-100%
	Negative Predictive Value	24-91%	40-100%	52-100%
	Positive Predictive Value	70-98%	69-96%	86-100%
	Accuracy	65-93%	73-97%	85-100%

Table 4. Diagnostic Performance of Endoscopic Ultrasound with and without Fine Needle Aspiration in Comparison to Computerized Tomography for Pancreatic Cancers in the Presence and Absence of Obstructive Jaundice

5.1 Cancer staging

The accuracy of EUS for the stage of patients with pancreatic cancer is superior to US and CT scans with values ranging between 85 and 100% in comparison to 64-66% for CT and 61-64% for US [55,71]. The EUS accuracy in staging pancreatic cancer does not depend on the use of radial or linear scanners [65]. Radial scanners offer a better overview of surrounding structures, whereas linear scanners allow the safe execution of tissue sampling. Initial studies showed excellent accuracy up to 94%, but later publication reported lower values ranging between 63% and 78% [55,72-76]. Overall, EUS-FNA is highly sensitive (84%), specific (97%), accurate (84%) and has a high positive predictive value (99%), but relatively low negative predictive value (64%)[77] (**Table 5**). A major problem in staging pancreatic cancer is the prediction of resectability as the best chance for long-term survival occurs in patients with localized disease undergoing resection. The primary goal of surgical therapy is to achieve a margin-negative R0 resection with minimal postoperative complications and a secondary important goal is to avoid unnecessary laparotomies for unresectable tumors[78].

Combining the pre-operative utilization of CT and EUS proved to be the method with the highest accuracy compared to each single technique to predict tumor resectability[79].
In this context, a preoperative assessment of R0 resectability becomes critically important. Radiologic staging with EUS and CT or MRI is currently used to identify patients who may be resectable. The criteria of unresectability of pancreatic cancer include evidence of distant metastasis, tumor enchroachment (defined as tumor surrounding the vessel more than 180 degrees) of arteries such as the celiac artery, hepatic artery, superior mesenteric artery (SMA) or massive venous invasion with thrombosis. Portal or superior mesenteric venous invasion without thrombosis or obliteration of vessels can still be classified as resectable tumors. A recent study comparing the roles of EUS, CT, MRI and angiography in the assessment of pancreatic cancer staging and respectability, has shown that CT scan was the most accurate in assessing the stage of the tumor (73%), locoregional invasion (74%), vascular involvement (83%), distant metastases (88%), final TNM stage (46%) and overall tumor resectablity (83%) [76]. Although EUS appeared to be superior to detect smaller tumors not visualized by CT scan it is important to recognize that most surgeons would probably not rely on EUS alone before making important therapeutic decisions about surgical resections[80].

	No Discrete Mass on CT		Discrete Mass on CT Scan	
	EUS	EUS-FNA	EUS	EUS-FNA
Sensitivity	82-100%	65-99%	93-100%	77-96%
Specificity	29-96%	59-100%	0-71%	29-100%
Negative Predictive Value	48-100%	40-97%	na	7-70%
Positive Predictive Value	68-99%	79-100%	85-99%	92-100%
Accuracy	63-99%	74-99%	85-99%	78-96%

Table 5. Diagnostic Value of Performing EUS-FNA Along with Spiral CT in Patients with Suspected Pancreatic Cancer

5.2 Conclusions
EUS-FNA has greatly impacted the diagnostic management of patients affected by pancreatic masses in conjunction with other cross sectional imaging tests. EUS is the best

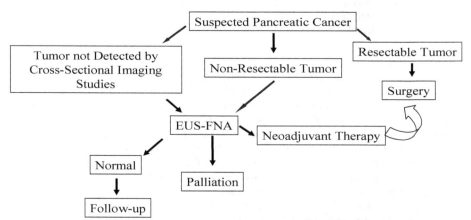

Fig. 1. Flow Chart for the Evaluation and Management of Patients with Suspected Pancreatic Malignancies

method for tissue diagnosis and it is extremely useful for the management of patients who are not surgical candidates and who require neo-adjuvant or palliative chemoradiation therapy. Conversely, pre-operative tissue diagnosis is not indispensable for resectable tumors and therefore EUS plays a lesser role in this group of patients. In recent years, EUS has assumed an important interventional role in the management of patients who are affected by debilitating pancreatic cancer pain as it is extremely useful in obtaining celiac plexus block for long term analgesic effects. Current role of EUS and EUS-FNA is summarized in **Figure 1**.

6. Pancreatic cystic lesions

Pancreatic cystic lesions (PCLs) are commonly identified due to increased use of cross-sectional imaging in patients with non-specific abdominal complaints. Although their exact prevalence is unknown, it is estimated to range from 1% to 2.6% of the general population based on large scale observational imaging studies using MDCT[81,82]. Pancreatic cystic lesions are strongly associated with increasing age and Asian race[82]. Their relative frequency varies substantially geographically and by institution (primary vs. secondary) due to different practices and patient populations [83]. In addition, the prevalence of PCLs including intraductal papillary mucinous neoplasms (IPMNs) was found to be higher among patients on hemodialysis compared to the normal population [84].

Inflammatory pseudocysts represent about 75% of pancreatic cysts; however they are not classified as true PCLs since they are non-epithelial inflammatory fluid collections associated with acute or chronic pancreatitis [85]. Based on surgical pathology, PCLs are classified according to the characteristics of the cells lining the cyst in benign, premalignant and malignant [86](**Table 6**).

Serous cystadenomas (SCAs), mucinous cystadenocarcinomas (MCAs) and IPMNs represent 90% of PCLs and only the mucin producing neoplasms have been described to have risk of malignancy [87]. In a small percentage of patients, solid malignant tumors such as adenocarcinoma, neuroendocrine tumors and other less common causes can present with cystic degeneration [88].

6.1 Limitations of radiological imaging modalities for the diagnosis of PCLs

Trans-abdominal ultrasound (US) is a safe and cheap diagnostic modality that can be used to diagnose PCLs, however, its sensitivity and specificity are often affected by the operator's experience and the technical characteristics of the machine [89]. In addition, the deep position of the pancreas and the interposition of other organs such as the stomach and the transverse colon limit the capacity of US to identify small PCLs. The overall sensitivity of US in detecting pancreatic lesions ranges from 48% [8] to 89% [20].

The majority of studies describing the role of CT and MRI in the diagnosis of PCLs have been small and retrospective. Relying on radiological characteristics alone can be misleading, with up to 40% of serous and mucinous lesions being misdiagnosed as pseudocysts [85,90]. Reported overall diagnostic accuracy for these lesions has been highly variable ranging between 20% and 83% [91-93]. (**Table 7**)

In a large group of patients, accurate preoperative diagnosis of PCLs was reported in 20% for serous cystadenoma, 30% for mucinous cystadenoma and 29% for mucinous cystadenocarcinoma, as the majority of these lesions were misdiagnosed as pseudocysts [92]. MRI is equal or slightly superior to CT in diagnosing PCLs except in its limited ability to demonstrate calcifications in the tumor wall or septa [94].

Pseudocysts (no epithelial lining)
Conventional pseudocysts
Paraduodenal wall cyst (cystic dystrophy)
Infection-related pseudocysts

Cysts with mucinous epithelium
Intraductal papillary mucinous neoplasms
Intraductal oncocytic papillary neoplasms
Mucinous cystic adenoma
Mucinous cystic adenocarcinoma
Mucocele
Retention cysts

Serous (clear-cell) cystic tumors
Serous cystadenoma
VHL-associated pancreatic cysts
Serous cystadenocarcinomas (Extremely rare, case reports)

Squamous-lined cysts
Lymphoepithelial cysts
Epidermoid cysts within intrapancreatic accessory spleen
Dermoid cysts
Squamoid cyst of pancreatic ducts

Cysts lined by acinar cells
Acinar cell cystadenocarcinomas
Acinar cell cystadenomas (cystic acinar transformation)

Endothelial-lined cysts
Lymphangiomas

Degenerative or necrotic changes in solid tumors
Solid-pseudopapillary tumor
Cystic change in ordinary ductal adenocarcinoma
Cystic pancreatic endocrine neoplasia (islet cell tumors)
Cystic mesenchymal neoplasms

Other rare cystic lesions
Cystic hamartomas
Endometriotic cyst
Metastatic cystic neoplasms
Congenital or developmental cysts
Others

VHL= Von Hippel-Lindau

Table 6. Pancreatic cystic lesions classified by cells lining the cavity

For IPMN, magnetic resonance cholangiopancreatography (MRCP) seems to be superior to endoscopic retrograde cholangiopancreatography (ERCP) in detecting cysts communicating with the main pancreatic duct [95].

6.2 Endoscopic ultrasonography

Endoscopic ultrasound (EUS) allows high resolution imaging of the pancreas with the ability to provide fine morphological details. The combination of fine-needle aspiration (FNA) cytology with the other recently available diagnostic markers has further increased its diagnostic accuracy[96]. Indications for EUS-FNA should be considered based on diagnostic accuracy of alternative modalities, costs, patient comfort and safety [97] and should be performed only when the information obtained has the potential to alter patient's management [98]. EUS-FNA should not be performed when there is inability to clearly visualize the target lesion, presence of large vessels interposed in the path between the needle and the lesion, bleeding diathesis and for patients at high risk of tumor seeding [98] such as those with cholangiocarcinoma who are considered for liver transplantation [99]. Once a cystic lesion is identified, the main clinical issue is the characterization and eventual therapeutic approach. Diagnostic accuracy of EUS imaging alone for differentiating malignant versus premalignant or benign lesions is ranging between 82% and 96% [100-103].

The endosonographic features suggestive of malignancy are: wall thickness of 3 mm or greater, macroseptations with cystic compartments greater than 10 mm, presence of a mass or intramural growth or cystic dilation of the main pancreatic duct. These features have a sensitivity of 91%, a specificity of 60% and an accuracy of 72% in predicting malignant or potentially malignant PCLs [104]. The sensitivity, specificity, positive predictive value (PPV), negative predictive value (NPV) and accuracy of EUS in comparison to other imaging modalities is summarized in **Table 7**

Despite EUS alone is a very sensitive test, EUS-guided fine needle aspiration (FNA) provides additional information for the characterization of PCLs. In a study by Frossard et al., the results of EUS and EUS guided FNA were compared with the final surgical pathology report. The sensitivity, specificity, PPV and NPV of EUS-guided FNA in this study were 97%, 100%, 100% and 95% respectively[102]. On the other hand, corresponding values for EUS imaging alone were 71%, 30%, 49% and 40% respectively[102]. Yet, the overall sensitivity and accuracy of EUS-FNA cytology remains widely variable with average sensitivity and accuracy around 50% [62,103,112,113].

6.3 Cytology

The aspirated cyst fluid is generally analyzed for tumor markers, chemical and molecular analysis. Solid component associated with PCLs or regional lymph nodes can be aspirated for cytology or histology. EUS guided FNA is safe and rare complications include pancreatitis (2-3%), intracystic hemorrhage (<1%) and infection (<1%). The administration of antibiotic during the procedure is a common practice even if there are no data to support it [114]. Tumor cell seeding has been a significant concern; there is limited evidence on the actual rise of tumor spread by EUS-FNA [115]. Recent study has shown that EUS-FNA has a decreased risk of peritoneal tumor spread as compared with computed tomography-guided FNA (2.2% vs. 16.3%) [66]. During EUS-FNA, the operator should always avoid to insert the needle through malignant tissue to reach a suspicious lesion. An example of this may be a patient with gastric or esophageal cancer and a suspicious lymph node adjacent to the primary tumor as the needle would have tumor entrapped into the channel that could contaminate the final results.

Diagnostic modality	Author	Year	Sensitivity (%)	Specificity (%)	PPV (%)	NPV (%)	Accuracy (%)
US	Giovanni et al[8]	1994	48-95	40-91	92	100	46-64
	Bottger et al[20]	1998					
	Rosch et al[3]	1991					
	Niederau et al[105]	1992					
	Palazzo et al[21]	1993					
	Tanaka et al[106]	1996					
Doppler US	Candiani et al[107]	1998	50-94	80-100	79	88	81-95
	Casadei et al[23]	1998					
	calculli et al[108]	2002					
EUS	Akahoshi et al[72]	1998	98	97	94	100	90
	Sedlack et al[104]	2002					
	Legmann et al[55]	1998					
Contrast enhanced US	Dietrich et al[109]	2008	90	100	100	86	93
CT	Bronstein et al[26]	2004	77	100	na	na	73
	Megibow et al[27]	1995					
MDCT	Park et al[110]	2009	83-91	63-75	80	87	85-95
	Vargas et al[30]	2004					
	Diehl et al[31]	1998					
	Schima et al[33]	2002					
MRI-MRCP	Anderssonet al[37]	2005	83-92	63-85	95	79	89
PET	Maemura et al[38]	2006	87-100	67-77	94	100	85-95
	Delbeke et al[111]	1999					

Abbreviations: Ultrasound (US), Endoscopic ultrasound (EUS), Computed tomography (CT), Multi detector computed tomography (MDCT), Positron emission tomography (PET)

Table 7. Summary of the performance characteristics of imaging tests for the diagnosis of pancreatic cancer

6.4 Cystic fluid markers

Several markers can be measured in the fluid aspirated from the pancreatic lesions during EUS to differentiate mucinous from non mucinous cysts. The most commonly used are; CEA, carbohydrate antigen (CA) 19-9, CA 72-4, and CA 15-3 [116]. CEA appears be the most useful as levels higher than 192 ng/ml had an accuracy of 79% for mucinous lesion characterization and was superior to cytology and EUS morphology [103].

Other markers such as amylase and lipase are important in the evaluation of cystic pancreatic lesions. Amylase is usually elevated in inflammatory cysts like pseudocysts but also in IPMN due to communication between the cystic lesion and the pancreatic duct. Amylase level less than 250 U/L favors the diagnosis of benign or malignant cystic neoplasms versus pancreatic pseudocysts (sensitivity 44%, specificity 98%) [117].

Molecular markers are recently considered a more reliable alternative. A multicenter study on pancreatic cyst fluid DNA analysis demonstrated a strong association of mucinous cystic neoplasms with K-ras mutations occurring with other loss of heterozygosity (LOH) mutations[118]. Shen et al [119] assessed the correlation between this molecular diagnosis with a clinical consensus diagnosis for PCLs defined by histology, malignant cytology, or two concordant tests (such as EUS, cytology, or CEA>_192 ng/ml for mucinous cysts). The study showed that the two diagnostic methods correlated well and molecular analysis of pancreatic cyst fluid added diagnostic value to the preoperative diagnosis.

7. Conclusion

Pancreatic cystic lesions are detected more frequently than in the past due to more sensitive imaging modalities. The differentiation between benign and malignant cystic lesions is often challenging. EUS and EUS-FNA have become a leading modality for the differential diagnosis of these lesions as it provides imaging characteristics and the possibility of obtaining cytology or fluid samples with high sensitivity and specificity. Characterization of cystic morphology by other imaging studies should be supplemented by EUS-FNA as cytology, tumor markers and DNA analysis can further characterize these lesions and increase the diagnostic accuracy of premalignant and malignant cysts.

8. Summary

Despite the advancement of other cross sectional imaging tests, EUS appears to have a higher sensitivity in detecting small pancreatic neoplasms in comparison to CT. On the other hand EUS does not appear to be accurate enough in assessing the invasion of SMA and SMV and respectability of locally advanced tumors. Recent studies have shown improved diagnostic performance of EUS with the use of parenteral contrast agents and EUS-FNA plays a key role when. tissue diagnosis is needed.

9. References

[1] DiMagno EP, Buxton JL, Regan PT, et al. Ultrasonic endoscope. Lancet 1980;1:629-31.

[2] Yasuda K, Mukai H, Cho E, Nakajima M, Kawai K. The use of endoscopic ultrasonography in the diagnosis and staging of carcinoma of the papilla of Vater. Endoscopy 1988;20 Suppl 1:218-22.

[3] Rosch T, Lorenz R, Braig C, et al. Endoscopic ultrasound in pancreatic tumor diagnosis. Gastrointest Endosc 1991;37:347-52.

[4] Vilmann P, Hancke S. [Endoscopic ultrasound scanning of the upper gastrointestinal tract. Preliminary results]. Ugeskr Laeger 1991;153:422-5.

[5] Bhutani MS, Hawes RH, Baron PL, et al. Endoscopic ultrasound guided fine needle aspiration of malignant pancreatic lesions. Endoscopy 1997;29:854-8.

[6] Chang KJ, Katz KD, Durbin TE, et al. Endoscopic ultrasound-guided fine-needle aspiration. Gastrointest Endosc 1994;40:694-9.

[7] Gress FG, Savides TJ, Sandler A, et al. Endoscopic ultrasonography, fine-needle aspiration biopsy guided by endoscopic ultrasonography, and computed tomography in the preoperative staging of non-small-cell lung cancer: a comparison study. Ann Intern Med 1997;127:604-12.

[8] Giovannini M, Seitz JF. Endoscopic ultrasonography with a linear-type echoendoscope in the evaluation of 94 patients with pancreatobiliary disease. Endoscopy 1994;26:579-85.

[9] Chang KJ, Nguyen P, Erickson RA, Durbin TE, Katz KD. The clinical utility of endoscopic ultrasound-guided fine-needle aspiration in the diagnosis and staging of pancreatic carcinoma. Gastrointest Endosc 1997;45:387-93.

[10] Santo E. Pancreatic cancer imaging: which method? JOP 2004;5:253-7.

[11] Jemal A, Siegel R, Ward E, Hao Y, Xu J, Thun MJ. Cancer statistics, 2009. CA Cancer J Clin 2009;59:225-49.

[12] Lynch SM, Vrieling A, Lubin JH, et al. Cigarette smoking and pancreatic cancer: a pooled analysis from the pancreatic cancer cohort consortium. Am J Epidemiol 2009;170:403-13.

[13] Hassan MM, Bondy ML, Wolff RA, et al. Risk factors for pancreatic cancer: case-control study. Am J Gastroenterol 2007;102:2696-707.

[14] Iodice S, Gandini S, Maisonneuve P, Lowenfels AB. Tobacco and the risk of pancreatic cancer: a review and meta-analysis. Langenbecks Arch Surg 2008;393:535-45.

[15] Permert J, Ihse I, Jorfeldt L, von Schenck H, Arnqvist HJ, Larsson J. Pancreatic cancer is associated with impaired glucose metabolism. Eur J Surg 1993;159:101-7.

[16] Shaib YH, Davila JA, El-Serag HB. The epidemiology of pancreatic cancer in the United States: changes below the surface. Aliment Pharmacol Ther 2006;24:87-94.

[17] Sharma C, Eltawil KM, Renfrew PD, Walsh MJ, Molinari M. Advances in diagnosis, treatment and palliation of pancreatic carcinoma: 1990-2010. World J Gastroenterol 2011;17:867-97.

[18] Sener SF, Fremgen A, Menck HR, Winchester DP. Pancreatic cancer: a report of treatment and survival trends for 100,313 patients diagnosed from 1985-1995, using the National Cancer Database. J Am Coll Surg 1999;189:1-7.

[19] Gandolfi L, Torresan F, Solmi L, Puccetti A. The role of ultrasound in biliary and pancreatic diseases. Eur J Ultrasound 2003;16:141-59.

[20] Bottger TC, Boddin J, Duber C, Heintz A, Kuchle R, Junginger T. Diagnosing and staging of pancreatic carcinoma-what is necessary? Oncology 1998;55:122-9.

[21] Palazzo L, Roseau G, Gayet B, et al. Endoscopic ultrasonography in the diagnosis and staging of pancreatic adenocarcinoma. Results of a prospective study with comparison to ultrasonography and CT scan. Endoscopy 1993;25:143-50.

[22] Baarir N, Amouyal G, Faintuch JM, Houry S, Huguier M. [Comparison of color Doppler ultrasonography and endoscopic ultrasonography for preoperative evaluation of the mesenteric-portal axis in pancreatic lesions]. Chirurgie 1998;123:445-9.

[23] Casadei R, Ghigi G, Gullo L, et al. Role of color Doppler ultrasonography in the preoperative staging of pancreatic cancer. Pancreas 1998;16:26-30.

[24] Tamm EP, Silverman PM, Charnsangavej C, Evans DB. Diagnosis, staging, and surveillance of pancreatic cancer. AJR Am J Roentgenol 2003;180:1311-23.

[25] Choi BI, Chung MJ, Han JK, Han MC, Yoon YB. Detection of pancreatic adenocarcinoma: relative value of arterial and late phases of spiral CT. Abdom Imaging 1997;22:199-203.

[26] Bronstein YL, Loyer EM, Kaur H, et al. Detection of small pancreatic tumors with multiphasic helical CT. AJR Am J Roentgenol 2004;182:619-23.

[27] Megibow AJ, Zhou XH, Rotterdam H, et al. Pancreatic adenocarcinoma: CT versus MR imaging in the evaluation of resectability--report of the Radiology Diagnostic Oncology Group. Radiology 1995;195:327-32.

[28] Gangi S, Fletcher JG, Nathan MA, et al. Time interval between abnormalities seen on CT and the clinical diagnosis of pancreatic cancer: retrospective review of CT scans obtained before diagnosis. AJR Am J Roentgenol 2004;182:897-903.

[29] Ohwada S, Ogawa T, Tanahashi Y, et al. Fibrin glue sandwich prevents pancreatic fistula following distal pancreatectomy. World J Surg 1998;22:494-8.

[30] Vargas R, Nino-Murcia M, Trueblood W, Jeffrey RB, Jr. MDCT in Pancreatic adenocarcinoma: prediction of vascular invasion and resectability using a multiphasic technique with curved planar reformations. AJR Am J Roentgenol 2004;182:419-25.

[31] Diehl SJ, Lehmann KJ, Sadick M, Lachmann R, Georgi M. Pancreatic cancer: value of dual-phase helical CT in assessing resectability. Radiology 1998;206:373-8.

[32] Lu DS, Reber HA, Krasny RM, Kadell BM, Sayre J. Local staging of pancreatic cancer: criteria for unresectability of major vessels as revealed by pancreatic-phase, thin-section helical CT. AJR Am J Roentgenol 1997;168:1439-43.

[33] Schima W, Fugger R, Schober E, et al. Diagnosis and staging of pancreatic cancer: comparison of mangafodipir trisodium-enhanced MR imaging and contrast-enhanced helical hydro-CT. AJR Am J Roentgenol 2002;179:717-24.

[34] Ichikawa T, Haradome H, Hachiya J, et al. Pancreatic ductal adenocarcinoma: preoperative assessment with helical CT versus dynamic MR imaging. Radiology 1997;202:655-62.

[35] Irie H, Honda H, Kaneko K, Kuroiwa T, Yoshimitsu K, Masuda K. Comparison of helical CT and MR imaging in detecting and staging small pancreatic adenocarcinoma. Abdom Imaging 1997;22:429-33.

[36] Romijn MG, Stoker J, van Eijck CH, van Muiswinkel JM, Torres CG, Lameris JS. MRI with mangafodipir trisodium in the detection and staging of pancreatic cancer. J Magn Reson Imaging 2000;12:261-8.

[37] Andersson M, Kostic S, Johansson M, Lundell L, Asztely M, Hellstrom M. MRI combined with MR cholangiopancreatography versus helical CT in the evaluation of patients with suspected periampullary tumors: a prospective comparative study. Acta Radiol 2005;46:16-27.

[38] Maemura K, Takao S, Shinchi H, et al. Role of positron emission tomography in decisions on treatment strategies for pancreatic cancer. J Hepatobiliary Pancreat Surg 2006;13:435-41.

[39] Higashi T, Saga T, Nakamoto Y, et al. Diagnosis of pancreatic cancer using fluorine-18 fluorodeoxyglucose positron emission tomography (FDG PET) --usefulness and limitations in "clinical reality". Ann Nucl Med 2003;17:261-79.

[40] Wakabayashi H, Nishiyama Y, Otani T, et al. Role of 18F-fluorodeoxyglucose positron emission tomography imaging in surgery for pancreatic cancer. World J Gastroenterol 2008;14:64-9.

[41] Reese SA, Traverso LW, Jacobs TW, Longnecker DS. Solid serous adenoma of the pancreas: a rare variant within the family of pancreatic serous cystic neoplasms. Pancreas 2006;33:96-9.

[42] Stern JR, Frankel WL, Ellison EC, Bloomston M. Solid serous microcystic adenoma of the pancreas. World J Surg Oncol 2007;5:26.

[43] Institute TUNC. Surveiilance Epidemiology and End Results (SEER) database. 2007. Available from: URL:http://seer.cancer.gov/. 2007.

[44] Buchler MW, Wagner M, Schmied BM, Uhl W, Friess H, Z'Graggen K. Changes in morbidity after pancreatic resection: toward the end of completion pancreatectomy. Arch Surg 2003;138:1310-4; discussion 5.

[45] Birkmeyer JD, Siewers AE, Finlayson EV, et al. Hospital volume and surgical mortality in the United States. N Engl J Med 2002;346:1128-37.

[46] Cameron JL, Riall TS, Coleman J, Belcher KA. One thousand consecutive pancreaticoduodenectomies. Ann Surg 2006;244:10-5.

[47] Sahani DV, Shah ZK, Catalano OA, Boland GW, Brugge WR. Radiology of pancreatic adenocarcinoma: current status of imaging. J Gastroenterol Hepatol 2008;23:23-33.

[48] Yamao K, Okubo K, Sawaka A, et al. Endolumenal ultrasonography in the diagnosis of pancreatic diseases. Abdom Imaging 2003;28:545-55.

[49] Moesinger RC, Talamini MA, Hruban RH, Cameron JL, Pitt HA. Large cystic pancreatic neoplasms: pathology, resectability, and outcome. Ann Surg Oncol 1999;6:682-90.

[50] Oberg K. Neuroendocrine gastrointestinal tumours. Ann Oncol 1996;7:453-63.

[51] Fritscher-Ravens A, Izbicki JR, Sriram PV, et al. Endosonography-guided, fine-needle aspiration cytology extending the indication for organ-preserving pancreatic surgery. Am J Gastroenterol 2000;95:2255-60.

[52] Baron PL, Kay C, Hoffman B. Pancreatic imaging. Surg Oncol Clin N Am 1999;8:35-58.

[53] Muller MF, Meyenberger C, Bertschinger P, Schaer R, Marincek B. Pancreatic tumors: evaluation with endoscopic US, CT, and MR imaging. Radiology 1994;190:745-51.

[54] Chang KJ. Endoscopic ultrasound-guided fine needle aspiration in the diagnosis and staging of pancreatic tumors. Gastrointest Endosc Clin N Am 1995;5:723-34.

[55] Legmann P, Vignaux O, Dousset B, et al. Pancreatic tumors: comparison of dual-phase helical CT and endoscopic sonography. AJR Am J Roentgenol 1998;170:1315-22.

[56] Mertz HR, Sechopoulos P, Delbeke D, Leach SD. EUS, PET, and CT scanning for evaluation of pancreatic adenocarcinoma. Gastrointest Endosc 2000;52:367-71.

[57] Bhutani MS, Gress FG, Giovannini M, et al. The No Endosonographic Detection of Tumor (NEST) Study: a case series of pancreatic cancers missed on endoscopic ultrasonography. Endoscopy 2004;36:385-9.

[58] Erickson RA, Sayage-Rabie L, Avots-Avotins A. Clinical utility of endoscopic ultrasound-guided fine needle aspiration. Acta Cytol 1997;41:1647-53.

[59] Barthet M, Portal I, Boujaoude J, Bernard JP, Sahel J. Endoscopic ultrasonographic diagnosis of pancreatic cancer complicating chronic pancreatitis. Endoscopy 1996;28:487-91.

[60] Binmoeller KF, Thul R, Rathod V, et al. Endoscopic ultrasound-guided, 18-gauge, fine needle aspiration biopsy of the pancreas using a 2.8 mm channel convex array echoendoscope. Gastrointest Endosc 1998;47:121-7.

[61] Gress F, Gottlieb K, Sherman S, Lehman G. Endoscopic ultrasonography-guided fine-needle aspiration biopsy of suspected pancreatic cancer. Ann Intern Med 2001;134:459-64.

[62] Wiersema MJ, Vilmann P, Giovannini M, Chang KJ, Wiersema LM. Endosonography-guided fine-needle aspiration biopsy: diagnostic accuracy and complication assessment. Gastroenterology 1997;112:1087-95.

[63] Erickson RA, Garza AA. Impact of endoscopic ultrasound on the management and outcome of pancreatic carcinoma. Am J Gastroenterol 2000;95:2248-54.

[64] Bhutani MS. Endoscopic ultrasonography in pancreatic disease. Semin Gastrointest Dis 1998;9:51-60.

[65] Gress F, Savides T, Cummings O, et al. Radial scanning and linear array endosonography for staging pancreatic cancer: a prospective randomized comparison. Gastrointest Endosc 1997;45:138-42.

[66] Micames C, Jowell PS, White R, et al. Lower frequency of peritoneal carcinomatosis in patients with pancreatic cancer diagnosed by EUS-guided FNA vs. percutaneous FNA. Gastrointest Endosc 2003;58:690-5.

[67] Hollerbach S, Klamann A, Topalidis T, Schmiegel WH. Endoscopic ultrasonography (EUS) and fine-needle aspiration (FNA) cytology for diagnosis of chronic pancreatitis. Endoscopy 2001;33:824-31.

[68] Hayashi Y, Nakazawa S, Kimoto E, Naito Y, Morita K. Clinicopathologic analysis of endoscopic ultrasonograms in pancreatic mass lesions. Endoscopy 1989;21:121-5.

[69] Canto MI, Goggins M, Hruban RH, et al. Screening for early pancreatic neoplasia in high-risk individuals: a prospective controlled study. Clin Gastroenterol Hepatol 2006;4:766-81; quiz 665.

[70] Canto MI, Goggins M, Yeo CJ, et al. Screening for pancreatic neoplasia in high-risk individuals: an EUS-based approach. Clin Gastroenterol Hepatol 2004;2:606-21.

[71] Rosch T, Braig C, Gain T, et al. Staging of pancreatic and ampullary carcinoma by endoscopic ultrasonography. Comparison with conventional sonography, computed tomography, and angiography. Gastroenterology 1992;102:188-99.

[72] Akahoshi K, Chijiiwa Y, Nakano I, et al. Diagnosis and staging of pancreatic cancer by endoscopic ultrasound. Br J Radiol 1998;71:492-6.

[73] Cannon ME, Carpenter SL, Elta GH, et al. EUS compared with CT, magnetic resonance imaging, and angiography and the influence of biliary stenting on staging accuracy of ampullary neoplasms. Gastrointest Endosc 1999;50:27-33.

[74] Ahmad NA, Lewis JD, Ginsberg GG, Rosato EF, Morris JB, Kochman ML. EUS in preoperative staging of pancreatic cancer. Gastrointest Endosc 2000;52:463-8.

[75] Meining A, Dittler HJ, Wolf A, et al. You get what you expect? A critical appraisal of imaging methodology in endosonographic cancer staging. Gut 2002;50:599-603.

[76] Soriano A, Castells A, Ayuso C, et al. Preoperative staging and tumor resectability assessment of pancreatic cancer: prospective study comparing endoscopic ultrasonography, helical computed tomography, magnetic resonance imaging, and angiography. Am J Gastroenterol 2004;99:492-501.

[77] Eloubeidi MA, Chen VK, Eltoum IA, et al. Endoscopic ultrasound-guided fine needle aspiration biopsy of patients with suspected pancreatic cancer: diagnostic accuracy and acute and 30-day complications. Am J Gastroenterol 2003;98:2663-8.

[78] Bao PQ, Johnson JC, Lindsey EH, et al. Endoscopic ultrasound and computed tomography predictors of pancreatic cancer resectability. J Gastrointest Surg 2008;12:10-6; discussion 6.

[79] Helmstaedter L, Riemann JF. Pancreatic cancer--EUS and early diagnosis. Langenbecks
     Arch Surg 2008;393:923-7.
[80] Hartwig W, Schneider L, Diener MK, Bergmann F, Buchler MW, Werner J. Preoperative
     tissue diagnosis for tumours of the pancreas. Br J Surg 2009;96:5-20.
[81] Spinelli KS, Fromwiller TE, Daniel RA, et al. Cystic pancreatic neoplasms: observe or
     operate. Ann Surg 2004;239:651-7; discussion 7-9.
[82] Laffan TA, Horton KM, Klein AP, et al. Prevalence of unsuspected pancreatic cysts on
     MDCT. AJR Am J Roentgenol 2008;191:802-7.
[83] Volkan Adsay N. Cystic lesions of the pancreas. Mod Pathol 2007;20 Suppl 1:S71-93.
[84] Ishikawa T, Takeda K, Itoh M, et al. Prevalence of pancreatic cystic lesions including
     intraductal papillary mucinous neoplasms in patients with end-stage renal disease
     on hemodialysis. Pancreas 2009;38:175-9.
[85] Warshaw AL, Rutledge PL. Cystic tumors mistaken for pancreatic pseudocysts. Ann
     Surg 1987;205:393-8.
[86] Kloppel G, Luttges J. WHO-classification 2000: exocrine pancreatic tumors. Verh Dtsch
     Ges Pathol 2001;85:219-28.
[87] Friedel DM, Abraham B, Georgiou N, Stavropoulos SN, Grendell JH, Katz DS.
     Pancreatic cystic neoplasms. South Med J;103:51-7.
[88] Bose D, Tamm E, Liu J, et al. Multidisciplinary management strategy for incidental
     cystic lesions of the pancreas. J Am Coll Surg;211:205-15.
[89] Karlson BM, Ekbom A, Lindgren PG, Kallskog V, Rastad J. Abdominal US for diagnosis
     of pancreatic tumor: prospective cohort analysis. Radiology 1999;213:107-11.
[90] Mathieu D, Guigui B, Valette PJ, et al. Pancreatic cystic neoplasms. Radiol Clin North
     Am 1989;27:163-76.
[91] Le Borgne J, de Calan L, Partensky C. Cystadenomas and cystadenocarcinomas of the
     pancreas: a multiinstitutional retrospective study of 398 cases. French Surgical
     Association. Ann Surg 1999;230:152-61.
[92] Procacci C, Biasiutti C, Carbognin G, et al. Characterization of cystic tumors of the
     pancreas: CT accuracy. J Comput Assist Tomogr 1999;23:906-12.
[93] Bassi C, Salvia R, Molinari E, Biasutti C, Falconi M, Pederzoli P. Management of 100
     consecutive cases of pancreatic serous cystadenoma: wait for symptoms and see at
     imaging or vice versa? World J Surg 2003;27:319-23.
[94] Minami M, Itai Y, Ohtomo K, Yoshida H, Yoshikawa K, Iio M. Cystic neoplasms of the
     pancreas: comparison of MR imaging with CT. Radiology 1989;171:53-6.
[95] Koito K, Namieno T, Ichimura T, et al. Mucin-producing pancreatic tumors: comparison
     of   MR   cholangiopancreatography   with   endoscopic   retrograde
     cholangiopancreatography. Radiology 1998;208:231-7.
[96] Adler DG, Jacobson BC, Davila RE, et al. ASGE guideline: complications of EUS.
     Gastrointest Endosc 2005;61:8-12.
[97] Mizuno N, Bhatia V, Hosoda W, et al. Histological diagnosis of autoimmune
     pancreatitis using EUS-guided trucut biopsy: a comparison study with EUS-FNA. J
     Gastroenterol 2009;44:742-50.
[98] Hawes RH. Indications for EUS-directed FNA. Endoscopy 1998;30 Suppl 1:A155-7.
[99] Rosen CB, Heimbach JK, Gores GJ. Liver transplantation for cholangiocarcinoma.
     Transpl Int;23:692-7.

[100] Ahmad NA, Kochman ML, Lewis JD, Ginsberg GG. Can EUS alone differentiate between malignant and benign cystic lesions of the pancreas? Am J Gastroenterol 2001;96:3295-300.

[101] Ahmad NA, Kochman ML, Brensinger C, et al. Interobserver agreement among endosonographers for the diagnosis of neoplastic versus non-neoplastic pancreatic cystic lesions. Gastrointest Endosc 2003;58:59-64.

[102] Frossard JL, Amouyal P, Amouyal G, et al. Performance of endosonography-guided fine needle aspiration and biopsy in the diagnosis of pancreatic cystic lesions. Am J Gastroenterol 2003;98:1516-24.

[103] Brugge WR, Lewandrowski K, Lee-Lewandrowski E, et al. Diagnosis of pancreatic cystic neoplasms: a report of the cooperative pancreatic cyst study. Gastroenterology 2004;126:1330-6.

[104] Sedlack R, Affi A, Vazquez-Sequeiros E, Norton ID, Clain JE, Wiersema MJ. Utility of EUS in the evaluation of cystic pancreatic lesions. Gastrointest Endosc 2002;56:543-7.

[105] Niederau C, Grendell JH. Diagnosis of pancreatic carcinoma. Imaging techniques and tumor markers. Pancreas 1992;7:66-86.

[106] Tanaka S, Kitamra T, Yamamoto K, et al. Evaluation of routine sonography for early detection of pancreatic cancer. Jpn J Clin Oncol 1996;26:422-7.

[107] Candiani F, Meduri F, Norberto L, Calderone M. [Contrast media in ultrasonography. Venous involvement in tumors of the head of the pancreas]. Radiol Med 1998;95:29-33.

[108] Calculli L, Casadei R, Amore B, et al. The usefulness of spiral Computed Tomography and colour-Doppler ultrasonography to predict portal-mesenteric trunk involvement in pancreatic cancer. Radiol Med 2002;104:307-15.

[109] Dietrich CF, Braden B, Hocke M, Ott M, Ignee A. Improved characterisation of solitary solid pancreatic tumours using contrast enhanced transabdominal ultrasound. J Cancer Res Clin Oncol 2008;134:635-43.

[110] Park HS, Lee JM, Choi HK, Hong SH, Han JK, Choi BI. Preoperative evaluation of pancreatic cancer: comparison of gadolinium-enhanced dynamic MRI with MR cholangiopancreatography versus MDCT. J Magn Reson Imaging 2009;30:586-95.

[111] Delbeke D, Rose DM, Chapman WC, et al. Optimal interpretation of FDG PET in the diagnosis, staging and management of pancreatic carcinoma. J Nucl Med 1999;40:1784-91.

[112] Bruno M, Bosco M, Carucci P, et al. Preliminary experience with a new cytology brush in EUS-guided FNA. Gastrointest Endosc 2009;70:1220-4.

[113] Al-Haddad M, Gill KR, Raimondo M, et al. Safety and efficacy of cytology brushings versus standard fine-needle aspiration in evaluating cystic pancreatic lesions: a controlled study. Endoscopy;42:127-32.

[114] Jacobson BC, Baron TH, Adler DG, et al. ASGE guideline: The role of endoscopy in the diagnosis and the management of cystic lesions and inflammatory fluid collections of the pancreas. Gastrointest Endosc 2005;61:363-70.

[115] Shah JN, Fraker D, Guerry D, Feldman M, Kochman ML. Melanoma seeding of an EUS-guided fine needle track. Gastrointest Endosc 2004;59:923-4.

[116] Repak R, Rejchrt S, Bartova J, Malirova E, Tycova V, Bures J. Endoscopic ultrasonography (EUS) and EUS-guided fine-needle aspiration with cyst fluid analysis in pancreatic cystic neoplasms. Hepatogastroenterology 2009;56:629-35.

[117] van der Waaij LA, van Dullemen HM, Porte RJ. Cyst fluid analysis in the differential diagnosis of pancreatic cystic lesions: a pooled analysis. Gastrointest Endosc 2005;62:383-9.

[118] Khalid A, Zahid M, Finkelstein SD, et al. Pancreatic cyst fluid DNA analysis in evaluating pancreatic cysts: a report of the PANDA study. Gastrointest Endosc 2009;69:1095-102.

[119] Shen J, Brugge WR, Dimaio CJ, Pitman MB. Molecular analysis of pancreatic cyst fluid: a comparative analysis with current practice of diagnosis. Cancer 2009;117:217-27.

4

Laparoscopy in Diagnosis and Treatment of Small Bowel Diseases

Coco Claudio, Rizzo Gianluca, Verbo Alessandro,
Mattana Claudio, Pafundi Donato Paolo and Manno Alberto
Catholic University of the Sacred Hearth
Department of Surgical Sciences Rome
Italy

1. Introduction

Laparoscopy is defined as the technique of examining the abdominal cavity and its contents by creating a pneumoperitoneum. The first description of a laparoscopic approach goes back to 1901, by Kelling, who showed on a dog model that it was possible to look inside the abdomen by introducing a cystoscope after high-pressure insufflation (Kelling, 1901). The development of the technique over the next 50 years, passed through the creation of specific instruments that made easier accurate and complete examination of the peritoneal cavity, such as the Verres needle, first described to create pneumothorax for treating tuberculosis but successfully used in 1937 for the induction of the pneumoperitoneum (Veress, 1938) and the Hasson trocar (Hasson, 1974). In September 1985 Erich Muhe performed the first laparoscopic cholecystectomy in humans (Litynski, 1998). Muhe used a Veress needle to create a pneumoperitoneum, introduced a laparoscope through the umbilicus, and completed laparoscopic cholecystectomy in 2 hours. The technique was presented at the Annual Congress of the German Surgical Society held in Munich on April 1986, and rapidly became the gold standard in the treatment of symptomatic gallstones. Fast and worldwide success of laparoscopic cholecistectomy was based on the analysis of results in terms of hospitalization, bowel function resumption, wound-related complications and return to daily activities, which were much more satisfying as compared to those obtained with the open technique, thus causing rapid acceptance by surgeons and increasing demand by patients. The laparoscopic approach was widely applied in abdominal surgery, for the treatment of a great number of benign disease, from MRGE to hernia, and even to procedures in which dissection and extraction of solid organs was contemplated, as safe and easy techniques rapidly developed. This affected transplantation surgery in the way that people who accept to donate the kidney rapidly increased after the diffusion of the laparoscopic approach, because of the decreased morbidity of the operation. Although first met with skepticism, laparoscopy have been applied to malignancies, especially to colon cancer. Many multicenter prospective randomized trials comparing laparoscopic and open technique in colon cancer surgery, unequivocally demonstrated the same favorable short term results of laparoscopic colectomy shown when this approach was adopted for other benign diseases (less intra-operative bleeding, less post-operative pain, morbidity and immunological stress, early bowel movement, shorter hospital stay, early return to daily activities and better cosmetic results). The laparoscopic technique demonstrated also effective considering some pathological parameters of oncological radicality, as number of lymph node removed and cancer-free margins. Non differences about long-term results, in terms of incidence of recurrence and overall survival, were shown between open and laparoscopic approach in any prospective randomized trial (Nelson et al., 2004), Another area where laparoscopy found a place in the last two decades is bariatric surgery. This, in part, is because of the results of the laparoscopic Roux-en-Y gastric bypass procedure, especially the minimally invasive surgical benefits and the resolution of obesity-related comorbidities (Robinson et al., 2004). The Lap-Band (BioEnterics Lap-Band System; Inamed Health, Santa Barbara, CA) also has become a popular minimally invasive tool with less morbidity than the gastric bypass. Despite the improvement in outcomes with laparoscopy, the technique has limitations. The video images are projected in a 2-dimensional plane. The stability, focus and tilt depends on camera operator, and the ability to follow the natural movement of the surgeon's eyes is limited. The use of trocars anchored to the abdominal wall limits the range of motion of the long straight instruments and often induces awkward ergonomics (Ballantyne, 2002). This conditions, combined with the counteracting vectors generated by the abdominal wall (which require force to overcome), can lead to surgeon fatigue or, worse, neurapraxia. Another problem of laparoscopic technique is represented by the learning curve that must be substantial, especially for more complex procedures (Berguer, 1998; Ehrmantraut & Sardi, 1997).

2. General considerations about diagnostic and therapeutic potential of laparoscopy in small bowel diseases

Small bowel diseases are rare and difficult to identify with traditional diagnostic tools. Diagnosis is often late, based on the appearance of occult rectal bleeding, occlusive syndrome or, more rarely, intestinal perforation. The exact identification and location of small bowel lesions were made easier in recent years by the development of more detailed diagnostic tools, such as double balloon enteroscopy and videocapsula (Gerson, 2009). The laparoscopic approach to the small bowel diseases may include resection or not. Well recognized examples of the first group are benign or malignant tumours; inflammatory bowel disease; Meckel's diverticulum; bleeding small bowel angiodysplasia; small bowel ischemia and stricture (postradiation, postischemic, etc). Non resectional laparoscopic small bowel procedures include laparoscopic enterolysis for acute small bowel obstruction, diagnostic laparoscopy for possible ischemic disease and laparoscopic palliative enteroenterostomy for bypassing obstructing nonresectable tumors. When dealing with small bowel pathologies, performing laparoscopy may be extremely challenging, as a consequence of the technical difficulties in the mobilization of the intestinal loops, especially if dilated as a consequence of an occlusion, or in identifying and localizing the lesions. Many difficulties were recently overcome with the help of technological development of instrumentation, such as the laparoscopic model of Ultracision®, Harmonic scalpel® or Ligasure®, so that nowadays laparoscopic diagnosis and treatment of small bowel diseases are to be considered feasible (Carrasco Rojas, 2004), although not easy to perform. In addition, endoscopic tattooing of the lesion, can make location of tumors easier.

3. Small bowel neoplasms

Small bowel neoplasms represent 0.3% of all tumors, fewer than 2% of all gastrointestinal malignances, with an age-adjusted incidence of 1 per 100,000 and a prevalence of 0.6%. Approximately, almost forty different histological types of both benign and malignant tumors have been identified (Neugut et al., 1998). Seventy five percent of tumors are benign at histologic diagnosis by biopsy and include leiomyomas, adenomas, lipomas and hamartomas. Malignant neoplasms, frequently symptomatic, include adenocarcinomas, carcinoids and lymphomas. Stromal tumors are considered as tumors with variable malignant power. Other type of small bowel malignant neoplasms are metastatic diseases by malignant melanoma, bronchogenic tumors, breast cancer and intrabdominal cancers. Surgery, is considered the first line therapy for most of the small bowel neoplasm, especially malignant and complicated benign tumors (Gill et al., 2001; Coco et al. 2010). Laparoscopic surgery represents a valid and feasible approach for the treatment of these neoplasms.

3.1 Benign neoplasms

Benign neoplasms are usually asymptomatic and only incidentally discovered, when complicated by obstruction or hemorrhage (more frequently occult). Despite the term "benign", exists a risk of malignant change for adenomas (malignant changes at presentation over 40%, expecially in large adenomas with villous component or atypia,) and leyomiomas (risk for malignancy related to the tumor size and number of mitosis); because of their potential to undergo malignant transformation, these neoplasms should be removed (Witteman et al., 1993). Lipoma, hemangioma, Bunner's gland hamartoma and intestinal nodular lymphoid hyperplasia have no risk of malignant evolution and indication for surgery is limited to symptomatic lesions (intussusceptions, obstruption, bleeding) (Morgan et al., 2000). These neoplasm are often multiple; a carefully inspection of the entire small bowel is recommended before the treatment. Surgical options are different: endoscopic treatment (endoscopic polypectomy or mucosectomy especially for benign neoplasms of duodenum or proximal jejunum), excision via enterotomy (especially for small lesions) and small bowel segmentary resection. In the last two cases the laparoscopic approach is advisable not only becasuse the resection is safe and effective but also becasuse the mandatory examination of the entire small bowel can be performed acording to a mini-invasive approach which consent to avoid laparotomy for treating benign diseases.

3.2 Malignant neoplasms

A recent epidemiologic study concerning small bowel malignant neoplasm, conducted in the United States on 67843 patients from 1973 to 2005 by Bilimoria et al (Bilimoria et al 2009), showed an overall increase, in the last thirty years, of small bowel cancer (22.7 cases per million in 2004). In particular, the proportion of patients with carcinoid tumors increased significantly (from 27.5% to 44.3%) whereas the proportion of patients with adenocarcinoma decreased (from 42.1% to 32.6%). However, incidence rates is low and similar for both men and women before the age of 40. In the last 30 years, there is a parallel increase between 40 and 55 yrs in both sexes and a more rapidly growth in men than in women. The sites at major risk for malignant neoplasm are duodenum, for adenocarcinoma, and ileum, for carcinoids and lymphomas (Lepage et al., 2006). Treatment modality and oncologic outcome differs considering the various histological types.

3.2.1 Small bowel carcinoid

Small bowel, especially terminal ileum, represents the most frequent location of neuroendocrine tumors (Fig. 1) in the gastrointestinal tract (among 30%). Peak incidence is between the 6th and 7th decades of life. Clinical manifestations are vague or absent, and tumors are often incidentally detected at the time of surgery for other gastrointestinal diseases or during exploration for liver metastases. In approximately 20% of cases these neoplasms secrete bioactive mediators and give rise to the characteristic "carcinoid syndrome" (intermittent abdominal cramps, diarrhea, flushing, bronchospasm and cyanosis) (Kulke & Meyer, 1999).

Nodal metastases after carcinoids are frequent (over 40% of cases) with no relations to tumor's dimensions, whereas liver metastases are usually associated to tumors > 2 cm in diameter (over 60% of cases). Resection of primary tumor with associated extensive mesenteric lymphadenectomy is appropriate, even in the presence of liver metastases. If diagnosis of intestinal carcinoid tumor is made after a limited resection of a small lesion, further surgery for extensive mesenteric lymphadenectomy is to be considered (Sutton et al., 2003). The indications for potentially curative liver resection are similar to those applicable to metastatic colorectal cancer. Disease unsuitable for partial hepatectomy unresponsive to alternative therapies, producing life-threatening complications and carcinoids with low proliferation index could be considered for liver transplantation (Yao et al., 2001). After radical resection of carcinoid tumors the 5yr-OS is good, with an OS rate of 70-80% in case of localized disease, 60-75% in case of nodal involvement and 30-50% in case of liver metastases. In patients with liver metastases who underwent to hepatectomy or liver transplantation 5y-OS is respectively 70-80% and 60-70% (Shebani et al., 1999).

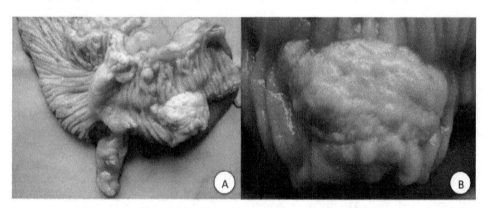

Fig. 1. A,B - Small bowel carcinoid

3.2.2 Small bowel adenocarcinoma

Adenocarcinoma (Fig. 2) represents the commonest histological type of small bowel tumors in the western world (30-50% of small bowel malignant tumors). Duodenum and jejunum are the most frequent location sites. Peak incidence is in the 7th decade of life and there is a male preponderance. Adenomas, either single or multiple as expression of multiple polyposis syndromes are to be considered lesions at risk of developing malignancies. Small bowel adenocarcinomas, because of the presence of lymphatic tissue in small intestinal mucosa, early metastasize to regional lymph node. The most common symptoms at presentation are obstruction, bleeding, jaundice and weight loss. Surgical radical resection followed by adjuvant chemotherapy represent the therapy of choice (Neugut et al., 1997). For jejunal and ileal tumors, curative resection (R0) is to be intended as complete removal of the neoplastic mass with macro- and microscopically clear margin and regional lymphnode dissection. If infiltration of continuous organs is detected, en bloc resection is indicated as well as right colectomy should be considered in case of distal ileal lesion, to obtain a complete nodal dissection. For duodenal tumors located in the II or III duodenal portions, duodenopacreatectomy is indicated, while for IV portion lesions, pancreas-preserving segmental resection will be the treatment of choice; in both cases clear resection margins are mandatory to obtain satisfing long term results. For locally advanced unresectable or metastatic adenocarcinoma a palliative treatment should be considered to avoid complication as obstruction (by-pass or stent) or bleeding (limited resection of the bleeding mass). In case of single hepatic metastasis, the role of liver resection is unknown (Hutchins et al., 2001). Despite radical resection, the 5yr-OS rate is low. In a large landmark study conducted by the American College of Surgeons Commission on 5,000 small bowel adenocarcinomas, the overall 5-year disease-specific survival was 30.5%, with a median survival of 19.7 months (Howe et al., 1999). Survival was lower in patients with duodenal tumors and in those over 75 years old, also because many surgeons are reluctant to perform radical resection in these cases (North & Pack, 2000).

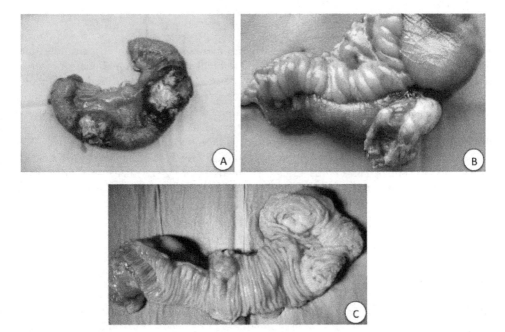

Fig. 2. A, B, C – Small bowel adenocarcinomas

3.2.3 Small bowel lymphoma

Small bowel lymphoma (Fig. 3) can be primary or secondary. Primary lymphoma accounts for 15% to 20% of all malignant small bowel tumors and ileum represents the most common location site. The usual clinical presentation of gastointestinal lymphoma includes intermittent abdominal pain, fatigue, diarrhea, weight loss, and, occasionally, fever; less commonly, gastrointestinal bleeding, obstruction, or even perforation (up to 25%). Chemoradiation is the therapy of choice for these neoplasms. In a clinical setting in which palpable adenopathy and hepatosplenomegaly are absent, with no evidence of disease on chest CT, diagnosis of primary intestinal lymphomas requires histologic confirmation. Only in this case, surgical exploration and resection of involved segments with regional lymph node dissection is requested to confirm diagnosis of lymphoma. Surgical treatment is required also in cases of complications as obstruction, bleeding and perforation. The overall prognosis of the more advanced stages of primary small intestinal lymphoma is poor, with an expected 5-year survival of 25% to 30% (Crump et al., 1999).

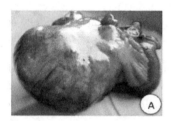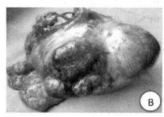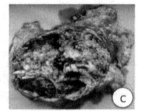

Fig. 3. A, B, C – Small bowel lymphomas

3.2.4 Small bowel stromal tumor

Stromal tumors account <1% of all gastrointestinal tumors. GISTs (Gastro Intestinal Stromal Tumors) represents the most common stromal tumors with malignant power of the gastrointestinal tract (over 90%) (Fig. 4). Many GISTs are discovered incidentally. When exist, symptoms of GISTs are obstruction, hemorrhage or, rarely, peritonitis. Malignant power of GIST depend by mitotic index and tumor size. Surgical complete gross resection with an intact pseudocapsule (non-disruptive techniques) and negative macroscopic margins (R0 or "R1" resection) is the definitive treatment for primary GISTs without evidence of peritoneal seeding or metastasis. En bloc resection is requested in case of infiltration of continuous organs (Demetri et al., 2004). Because GISTs rarely metastasize to lymph nodes, routine lymph node dissection is not warranted except when there is evidence of gross nodal involvement (Blay et al, 2005). In advanced cases surgery alone is not curative. Resection of intraperitoneal metastases should be considered if they are prone to intralesional bleeding, which may result in severe blood loss, peritonitis, and interference with Imatinib therapy but most metastatic lesions from GIST, particularly those to the liver, are multifocal, diffuse, and technically difficult to resect (Everett & Gutman, 2008). The 5-year survival rate after the surgical resection of GIST was 43–95% in the pre-Imatinib era variable from 95% for low-risk GISTs to 0%-30% for high-risk GISTs. After the introduction of molecular targeted therapy with Imatinib and Sunitinib improvement in survival seems to be granted, but most prospective randomized studies are needed.

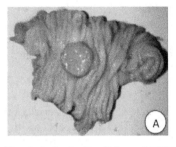
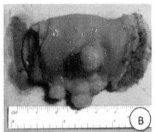
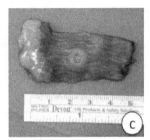

Fig. 4. A, B, C - Small bowel GISTs

3.2.5 Metastatic neoplasms

Secondary neoplastic involvement of the small intestine is more frequent than primary lesions. Primary tumors of colon, ovary, uterus, and stomach usually involve the small bowel, either by direct invasion or by intraperitoneal spread, whereas primaries of breast, lung, and melanoma, the malignancy which more frequently metastasize to the bowel, spread hematogenously. (Fig. 5). Surgical resection does not improve prognosis but is sometimes requested in case of complications.

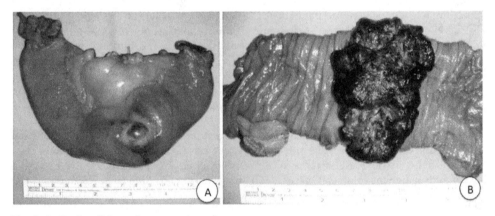

Fig. 5. A, B - Small bowel metastatic melanoma

3.2.6 Role of laparoscopic surgery

Among small bowel tumors, the mini-invasive approach is clearly accepted only for GISTs. The 2004 NCCN Task Force Report generally discouraged laparoscopic or laparoscopy-assisted resection for GIST, limiting its use for tumors smaller than 2 cm at low risk of intraoperative rupture (Demetri et al., 2004). However, two years later, Novitsky et al. (Novitsky et al., 2006) analyzing the results of their series of 50 laparoscopically operated GISTs of mean size of 4.4 cm (range, 1.0–8.5 cm), showed that efficacy and recurrence rate were similar or even better than what reported in historical open-surgery control series, and suggested a revision of the 2004 NCCN guidelines. So the 2007 update stated that laparoscopic resection was acceptable for tumors measuring up to 5 cm in diameter and that tumors larger than 5 cm might be resectable by hand-assisted laparoscopic techniques

(Demetri et al., 2004). Although there are no guidelines to state the feasibility of laparoscopic surgery for carcinoid, lymphoma, adenocarcinoma and other malignancies of the small intestine, we believe that this technique is feasible in these cases, especially with the help of the same useful devices used in laparoscopic colorectal cancer surgery (sterile drape ®, etc.).

4. Small bowel Crohn's disease

Crohn's disease (CD) is a common chronic inflammatory disease usually characterized by patchy, whole thickness, granulomatous lesions, that can affect any part of the gastrointestinal tract (Fig. 6). The incidence of CD is 5-10 per 100 000 per year with a prevalence of 50-100 per 100 000 (Carter et al., 2004). Clinical patterns include combined small and large intestinal pattern (26% to 48%), small intestine only pattern (11% to 48%) and colon only pattern (19% to 51%) (Munkholm & Binder, 2004). Involvement of terminal ileum and colon is the most common pattern (55%), while involvement of mouth, oesophagus, stomach and duodenum, is uncommon and rarely occurs without concurrent disease activity in the small bowel and/or colon (Thoreson & Cullen, 2007). Patients with small bowel CD commonly present with an acute symptomatic picture, characterized by abdominal cramps, diarrohea, malaise and loss of weight that is primarily managed using steroids, immunomodulators (Azathioprine, Mercaptopurine, Methotrexate) or biological therapy (anti-TNF agents) (Travis et al, 2006). Surgical treatment is required in approximately 70 percent of patients for failed medical therapy, recurrent intestinal obstruction, malnutrition and for septic complications (free perforation, abscess). Reoperations are required in 70 to 90 percent of all patients and multiple procedures in more than 30 percent (Duepree et al, 2002). Resection and anastomosis is indicated for short segment with multiple strictures or active disease, diseased bowel with fistula, abscess or phlegmon. Strictureplasty is a safe and effective alternative to bowel resection as multiple ones are often required for the same patient, with high risk of a short bowel syndrome.

Laparoscopy has gained wide acceptance in gastrointestinal surgery with potential advantages in early post-operative outcome and cosmesis (Duepree et al, 2002; Dunker et al, 1998; Milsom et al., 1993; Reissman et al, 1996; Albaz et al., 2000) and its use is accepted in benign and malignant colorectal diseases. The first laparoscopic intestinal resection for CD was reported by J. Milsom in 1993 (Milsom et al., 1993). Laparoscopic surgery offers additional advantage of smaller abdominal fascial wounds, low incidence of hernias, and decreased rate of adhesive small-bowel obstruction (Albaz et al., 2000) than conventional surgery. The main concerns about laparoscopic approach to small bowel CD are: missing occult segments of disease and critical proximal strictures due to absence of tactile sensitivity; earlier recurrence due to possible reduced immune response, technical difficulties due to fragile inflamed bowel and mesentery and the presence of adhesions, fistulas, and abscesses (Uchikoshi et al., 2004; Lowney et al., 2005). A Cochrane review about the role of laparoscopic surgery in CD was recently published (Bobby et al., 2011). Two randomized controlled trials (Maartense et al., 2006; Milsom et al., 2001) comparing laparoscopic and open surgery for small bowel CD were identified for a total of 120 patients. About post-operative morbidity less patients in the laparoscopic group (2/61; 3.27%) suffered wound infection compared to the open group (9/59; 15.25%) but the difference was not statistically significant (p=0.23). There was no significant difference in the incidence of other postoperative complications (postoperative pneumonia, prolonged postoperative ileus and urinary infections). The incidence of anastomotic leak, intra abdominal abscess and 30-day reoperation rates were comparable. The operation time was shorter in open surgery and the amount of intra operative blood loss was lesser in the open group (133 +/- 70 ml/case) compared to laparoscopic group (173 +/- 123 ml/case) although the difference was not statistically significant [P=0.25].. There was no significant difference in postoperatve pain as defined by the amount of opioids requested by patients. Hospital stay was shorter in laparoscopic group compared to open group but the difference was not statistically significant [P=0.90]. Conversion rates were similar in both the trials [3 out of 30 in Maartense 2006 and 2 out of 33 in Milsom 2001]. There was no significant difference in the reoperation rates for disease recurrence. Laparoscopic surgery for abdominal conditions is known to have associated with lesser incidence of adhesions and incisional hernias. Better cosmesis and body image obtained with the laparoscopic approach are well establisehd and are particularly relevant dealing with Crohn's disease, because of the young age of patients. Quality of Life (QoL) was not evaluated in this Cochrane review (Bobby et al., 2001), although a randomized control trial (Eshuis et al., 2010) reported similar QoL in both groups.

In conclusion, despite there are no potential benefits of laparoscopic surgery over open surgery, this approach for small bowel CD is feasible and as safe as the pen one, but with better cosmetic results and short-term post-operative outcome.

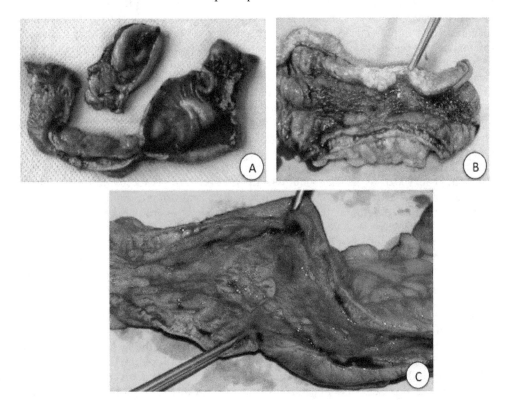

Fig. 6. A, B, C – Small bowel Crohn's Disease

5. Meckel's diverticulum

Meckel's diverticulum is the most common congenital malformation of the gastrointestinal tract (incidence of between 0.6% and 4%) due to persistence of the congenital vitello-intestinal duct. It is a true diverticulum, typically located on anti-mesenteric border, 60 cm from the ileo-caecal junction, and contains all three coats of intestinal wall with its separate blood supply from the vitelline artery. In the fetal life, the omphalo-mesenteric duct connects the yolk sac to the intestinal tract and usually it obliterates in the 5th to 7th week of life. If obliteration fails, the congenital anomalies develop, leading to residual fibrous cords, umbilical sinus, omphalo-mesenteric fistula, enterocyst and, most commonly, Meckel's diverticulum. The range of incidence of complications due to Meckel's diverticulum is 4%–16%. Its occurrence in males and females is equal, but incidence of complications is three to four times greater in males. The risk of complications decreases with increasing age, with no other predictive factors. Bleeding from Meckel's diverticulum due to ectopic gastric mucosa is the most common clinical presentation, especially in younger patients. The main mechanism of bleeding is the acid secretion from ectopic mucosa, leading to ulceration of adjacent ileal mucosa. It is possible that the recurrent intussusception may cause trauma, inflammation, mucosal erosion and bleeding. Others complications in adults include: obstruction, intussusceptions, ulceration and, rarely, vescico-diverticular fistulae and tumours (Heinicke et al., 1997; Wong et al., 2005; Tan et al., 2005; Puliglandla et al., 2001).

Due to the rarity of cases in adults, it is still misdiagnosed preoperatively. Preoperative diagnosis of symptomatic Meckel's diverticulum is difficult; so, it is imperative to differentiate Meckel's diverticulum from other surgical conditions. This is particularly true in patients presenting with symptoms other than bleeding. In a study by Higachi et al. about 776 patients affected by Meckel's diverticulum, a correct preoperative diagnosis was made in 88% of those presenting with bleeding but only in 11% of cases when other symptoms were reported (Higaki et al., 2001). In doubtful cases, laparoscopy is an excellent diagnostic tool (Shalaby et al., 2005). However, technetium-99m pertechnate scan is the most common and accurate non-invasive investigation performed for these cases. In children, it has a sensitivity of 80%–90%, a specificity of 95% and an accuracy of 90% (Kong et al., 1993) but in adults it is less reliable, with a sensitivity of 62.5%, a specificity of 9% and an accuracy of 46% (Lin et al., 2002). As the technetium-99m pertechnate scan is specific to ectopic gastric mucosa and not to Meckel's diverticulum, it may be positive in gut duplication cysts with ectopic gastric mucosa (Kumar et al., 2005). The false negative scans may be due to the rapid dilution of radioactive secondary to fast bleeding from the ectopic mucosa, impaired vascular supply or insufficient gastric mucosa. The false negatives are also more common in patients presenting with other symptoms than bleeding. Other diagnostic method suggested to supplement the Meckel's scan is angiography but it is usually negative unless the bleeding rate is 40.5 mL/min. The treatment of choice for symptomatic Meckel's diverticulum is surgical resection. It can be achieved either by diverticulectomy or by segmental bowel resection, especially when there is palpable ectopic tissue at the junction between diverticulum and intestinal wall, intestinal ischaemia or perforation. It has long been stated that the risk of developing complications following the incidental removal of Meckel's diverticulum can offset the potential benefits of this procedure (Leijonmarck et al., 1996) and the subject is still object of debate. Opponents to incidental diverticulectomy often cite Soltero and Bill (Soltero & Bill, 1976) who, in 1976, estimated that the life-time risk of complications from an untreated MD was 4.2%, decreasing this risk to zero with increasing age, and so incidental diverticulectomy was not advisable. Twenty years later, the results of a large population-based study in Olmsted County, Minnesota, provided data in support of prophylactic diverticulectomy (Cullen et al., 1994). This study reported a 6.4% cumulative rate of developing complications from untreated MD that required surgery over a life-time, especially in male patients up to 80 years of age. Diverticulectomy for complicated MD carried an operative mortality and morbidity of 2% and 12%, and a cumulative risk of long term complications of 7%. The corresponding rates for incidental diverticulectomy are 1%, 2% and 2%, respectively (Cullen et al. 1994). A subsequent report from the Mayo Clinic recommended MD resection only in male patients younger than 50 years of age, when the diverticulum length is greater than 2 cm, or when abnormal features are detected within the diverticulum: carcinoid tumors was found in 2.2% of the symptomatic patients and in 2.1% of the asymptomatic ones in this series (Park et al., 2005). More recently, however, a systematic review of the English literature on this subject shown that there is no compelling evidence to support prophylactic resection (Zani et al., 2008). In fact, resection of incidentally detected MD has a significantly higher early complication rate than that potentially occurring leaving the diverticulum in situ (5.3% vs 1.3%, $P < 0.0001$) (Cullen et al., 1994). With the advent of gastrointestinal stapling devices, excision has become safer, faster, and more efficient. Another advantage of stapling is that it closes the bowel lumen as it cuts, thereby completely reducing the chance of peritoneal contamination. The contraindications for stapler excision is a very broad-based or too short diverticula, because in these cases, the risk of including too much of the ileum during stapling or leaving behind part of the diverticulum is high. Another way to perform the excision is to exteriorize the diverticulum throgh a mini-laparotomy, resect it by stapler and close the enterotomy. It is of crucial importance that the direction of the staple line lies perpendicular to the longitudinal axis of the ileum so that the bowel lumen will not be compromised while the stapler is positioned at the base of the diverticulum. The reticulating head of the stapler is invaluable in these situations because it can be maneuvered precisely at the base of the diverticulum.

Laparoscopy was succesfully used to diagnose and treat patients with MD complicated by small bowel obstruction or bleeding caused by occult heterotopic gastric mucosa (Sanders, 1995; Rivas et al., 2003). Successful resection of a Meckel's diverticulum can also be accomplished through laparoscopy, using endostapling devices. The advantages and benefits of minimal access surgery can be truly appreciated in children with symptomatic Meckel's diverticulum. A recent study demonstrate that laparoscopic stapler resection of asymptomatic diverticulum during surgery for unrelated disease has been shown to produce no added morbidity (Ruh et al., 2010).

6. Small bowel angiodysplasia and management of obscure-occult gastrointestinal bleeding

Angiodysplasia (Fig. 7) is a vascular malformation that can be located in all gastrointestinal tract. When symptomatic, it causes gastrointestinal bleeding, frequently obscure and occult, and anemia. Small bowel cases are often difficult to localize because traditional endoscopic tools (EGDS and colonoscopy) are not helpful. (Sass et al., 2004; Bodner et al., 2005; Martinez-Ares et al., 2004). Small intestine enteroscopy (double-balloon enteroscopy) is the most specific method for diagnosis but its application is limited because it is a time-consuming procedure, causes great discomfort to the patient, is often complicated by bleeding and perforation and has high false positive rate (Nguyen et al., 2005; Keuchel &

Hagenmuller, 2005; Warneke et al., 2004; Hartmann et al., 2005; Ell et al., 2002; Jones et al., 2005; Lewis & Swain, 2002). Capsule endoscope is a valid diagnostic tool but histological diagnosis through biopsy and cannot be achieved (Hartmann et al., 2005; Ell et al., 2002; Jones et al., 2005; Lewis & Swain, 2002). During the active stage of small intestinal bleeding, selective angiography can find the contrast medium flowing from the lesion into the intestinal tract, showing local shadow with a slightly high density, and concomitant embolic treatment can be performed (Yamaguchi et al., 2003). Scintigraphy with 99mTc-sestamibi marks the eritrocytes and is sensitive to mild intestinal bleeding, while it has no diagnostic value in the resting phase of bleeding or when it is less than 0.05 mL/min (Rerksuppaphol et al., 2004). So, diagnosis of massive obscure gastro-intestinal bleeding is usually made by laparotomy, which is invasive with a false positive rate of 5%. Laparoscopy can clearly, directly and conveniently observe the whole intestinal serosa and mesentery (Ell et al., 2002; Rerksuppaphol et al., 2004; Lee et al., 2000; Abbas et al., 2001; Loh & Munro, 2003; Kok et al., 1998) so that many authors agree that it is a very promising tool in the diagnosis and treatment of acute massive small intestinal bleeding and can be used as a routine method (Ell et al., 2002; Rerksuppaphol et al., 2004; Abbas et al., 2001; Kok et al., 1998).

Laparoscopic exploration of small intestinal hemangiomas or vascular deformity should be extremely careful. The intestinal wall should be carefully explored for local prominence, pitting, overlapping and abnormal mensentery. The suspected bleeding segment should be palpated carefully with clamps to feel its hardness, flexibility, and activity. In case of active massive bleeding, intestinal peristalsis is active and blood often accumulates in the distal segment which is dark blue under laparoscope. In cases in which the bleeding site is not individuated by laparoscopy, perioperative enteroscopy generally allow to reach the goal (Ell et al., 2002; Lee et al., 2000; Loh & Munro, 2003; Kok et al., 1998).

After the bleeding site was found by laparoscopy, laparoscopy-assisted bowel resection and enteroanastomosis were performed, by exploratory incision about 5 cm in length at the umbilicus level on the midline. The resected part of the small intestine should be 5 cm longer than the bleeding site that may result in a fast and reliable excision with light contaminations in the abdominal cavity. Enterectomy and enteroanastomosis can be performed, sometimes, with laparoscopic technique (Rerksuppaphol et al., 2004; Lee et al., 2000; Abbas et al., 2001; Loh & Munro, 2003; Kok et al., 1998).

In conclusion, laparoscopy in diagnosis and treatment of massive small intestinal bleeding is a minimally invasive procedure with potentially grants less pain, short recovery time and definite therapeutic efficacy than open approach. Randomized studies are necessary.

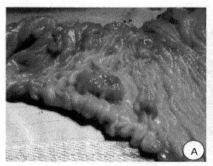 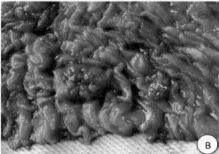

Fig. 7. A, B – Small bowel angiodysplasia

7. Other disease

Several other rare diseases which can cause obstruction (internal hernia, small bowel bezoar, intussusception, pseudo-obstruction) and bleeding (arteriovenous malformations, Delafoy's ulcer) are described in literature. In many of these cases laparoscopic surgery could represents a safe alternative to traditional open approach.

8. Adhesions and small bowel obstruction

Adhesions represent the most frequent cause of small bowel obstruction (SBO). Foster et al. in 2005, reported that in 1997, the 85% of the 32,583 unscheduled admissions for SBO in California were secondary to adhesions (Foster et al., 2006). In a recent Canadian study, of 552 patients admitted for SBO, 74% were secondary to adhesions (Miller et al., 2000). Treating adhesive SBO by surgery could seem a paradox because laparotomy is the most common cause of adhesive SBO. The cumulative recurrence rate of SBO after one open adhesiolysis for SBO is 7% at 1 year, 18% at 10 years, and 29% at 25 years. In patients who underwent a second open laparotomy for SBOs, recurrence rate is higher: 17% at 1 year, 32% at 10 years, and 40% at 20 years (Fevang et al., 2004). In the management of SBO conservative management is unanimously acccepted in the absence of signs of strangulation for a period varying from 12 hours to 5 days (Seror et al., 1993). CT scan is considered the ideal diagnostic tool to detect complicated SBO as it can show not only site, level and cause of obstruction but also sign of strangulation (Mak et al., 2006). About treatment of SBO two most large studies were performed. In the Canadian study by Foster et al (Foster et al., 2006) on 35,000 people admitted to the hospital for SBO, 75% were managed successfully conservatively with a 1-year mortality of 23% and 81% of surviving patients had no additional SBO readmissions over the subsequent 5 years. Small bowel obstruction was initially considered a condition not suitable for laparoscopy, as a consequence of the limited view of the abdominal cavity due to the dilated bowel, with high risk of accidental enterotomies. As surgeon's experience increased and better technological devices were produced, laparoscopic treatment of SBO became possible and it was rapidly evident that, in experienced hands, it could be a viable alternative to laparotomy as it allowed to decrease potential additional adhesions, together with the well known advantages of this approach. Selection criteria for laparoscopy (Duh, 1998) may be helpful: proximal obstruction, partial obstruction, anticipated single band, localized distension on radiography, no sepsis, and mild abdominal distension. A review published in 2007 show that laparoscopic management of SBO was successful in 66% of patients with a conversion rate of 33.5% (Ghosheh & Salameh, 2007) mostly due to dense adhesions (28%) followed by the need for bowel resection (23%) for injury, ischemia, gangrene, and other causes. The rate of success was significantly higher (p<0.001) in patients operated in the first 24 h and in patients with bands (54%), than in those with matted adhesions (31%). A recent review reported a morbidity rate of 15.5% and a mortality rate of 1.5% (Ghosheh & Salameh, 2007). Operative time longer than 120 minutes, intraoperative perforation, bowel necrosis, and conversion to laparotomy were significant predictors of post- operative morbidity (Strickland et al., 1999). Several animal studies (Riesman et al., 1996) supporting the hypothesis that laparoscopy leads to a decreased rate of adhesion formation as compared to laparotomy. This should be the main rationale to propose laparoscopy, rather than immediately recognizable benefits. It is not really clear, however, if laparoscopic adhesiolysis for SBO would lead to a decrease in recurrence rate. Ghosheh and Salameh (Ghosheh & Salameh, 2007) reported an early recurrence of SBO in 22 (2.1%) of 1,061 patients. However, no conclusion can be drawn regarding the true rate of recurrence of SBO since adequate follow-up is lacking in most of the published studies.

9. Surgical techniques

9.1 General principles

Mechanical bowel preparation antibiotic prophilaxis before laparoscopic surgery of the small bowel are the standard practice. Nasogastric tube and urinary catheter are commonly used, especially the last one as it is extremely useful in obtaining more space in the surgical field and decreasing chances of accidental injury by keeping the bladder empty during the procedure. The operation is performed under general anesthesia. The patient is positioned supine with tucked arms opened legs. The surgeon should stand facing the lesion: between the legs (our preferred position), on patient's right side, for lesions involving the proximal small bowel, or on the left side, for lesions involving the terminal ileum. The camera operator stands on surgeon's right side, if he is positioned between the legs of the patient or on the same side, if the surgeon is positioned laterally to the patient. The assistant stands on the opposite side of the operator. The surgeon should stand in line with the view of the laparoscope, with comfortable handling of ports and instruments with each hand. The monitor should be in front of the surgeon and facing the line of view of the telescope. The first trocar, used to introduce the laparoscope, should be placed in the umbilical region. Despite continuous evolution of both laparoscopic instruments and techniques, injuries to the intraabdominal structures are still a common complication of laparoscopy. Many of these injuries are related to the blind placement of the Veress needle or sharp first trocar into the abdomen,when performing the technique referred to as "closed" laparoscopy. Open laparoscopy, where the peritoneal cavity is opened before placing a blunt trocar into the abdomen, was then proposed and widely adopted, with remarkable success in avoiding major vessel injuries but not bowel ones. In response "optical-access" trocars were developed. These trocars were designed to decrease the risk of injury to intrabdominal structures by allowing the surgeon to visualize abdominal wall layers during placement. Two "optical-access" trocar systems are available: the first one uses a blade that strikes the fascia and peritoneum under laparoscopic visualization (Visiport, United States Surgical, Norwalk, CT), and the other one has a conical clear tip that is rotated under laparoscopic vision as it penetrates the fascia and peritoneum (Optiview, Ethicon Endo-Surgery, Cincinnati, OH). An angled (30- or 45-degree) camera gives the best view of the small bowel mesentery and is much preferred over a 0-degree scope. Additional trocars (5 mm or 10-12 mm, depending on instruments that will be used) are placed in the left and in the right abdomen, just below the level of the umbilicus. Other essential equipment includes atraumatic graspers for safely handling the bowel, laparoscopic scissors with attachment to monopolar cautery and laparoscopic intestinal staplers, both linear dividing (gastrointestinal anastomosis [GIA]-type) and linear closing (TA-type). Mesenteric section may be accomplished by using a combination of vascular endoscopic staplers, clips, or Ultracision Harmonic Scalpel® or Ligasure® which allow a proper dissection with minimal blood loss.

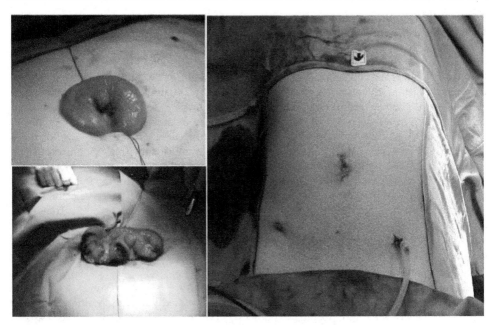

Fig. 8. Technical aspects of small bowel laparoscopic resection

Because of the potential for multifocal or unsuspected lesions, a careful exploration of the abdomen and all small bowel (from Treitz to ileo-cecal valve) is performed as the first step of the procedure, to exactly define the site and the extent of disease. Putting the patient on Trendelenburg position, the surgeon locates and grasps the transverse colon and maintains upward traction; then he changes the patient's position to reverse Trendelenburg, to slip down the small intestine away from the transverse colon, allowing identification of the Treitz ligament. The surgeon runs the small intestine between a pair of atraumatic clamps and identifies the segment that has to be resected. The location of the lesion will be more simple if previous spotting (during enteroscopy) has been performed. Adhesiolysis is often necessary. After identification and mobility evaluation of the small bowel tract involved by disease, a 4 cm midline peri-umbilical incision is performed, pneumoperitoneum is evacuated and the small bowel loop affected by disease, is pulled out from the abdominal cavity together with its mesentery (Fig. 8). Using a wound protection is mandatory if neoplasm is suspected. A V-shaped incision is performed on mesentery related to the small bowel loop affected by disease, using standard technique, and ligation of vascular pedicle is performed. Wide mesenteric excision is appropriate only when treating malignant lesions. The bowel is divided extracorporeally, by using an intestinal stapler. A mechanical or hand-sewn side-to-side or end-to-end anastomosis is usually performed extracorporeally. After performing the anastomosis, the mesenteric defect is closed (if possible) and the bowel is reintroduced into the abdominal cavity. After closure of the small incision and the reestablishment of the pneumoperitoneum, the surgeon must confirm hemostasis, and control the anastomosis. A para-anastomotic drainage is positioned using a trocar incision (Fig. 8). Mesenteric vessels ligation, bowel resection and anastomosis could also be performed intracorporeally.

9.2 Surgical techniques for small bowel resection for Crohn's disease

Under general anesthesia, the patient is placed in a supine position with both arms tucked at his or her sides. Three 5/10/12 mm trocars respectively, a 30° angled laparoscope and an intra-abdominal insufflation of 12 mmHg are used. The pneumoperitoneum is established following open Hasson trocar placement through an infraumbilical incision. Under laparoscopic vision, the other two trocars are placed in the patient's left flank, lateral to the rectus sheath. After a careful exploration of the abdomen to assess the site and extent of disease, the right colon, terminal ileum, and the inflammatory mass are fully mobilized, mainly with blunt dissection from the lateral to medial direction. The hepatic flexure is mobilized in most cases. No attempt should be made to transect the thick mesentery at this time. The right colon and the terminal ileum are extracted through a small (5−7 cm) right lower quadrant incision, using Pfannestiel or a midline incision. The terminal ileum and the cecum are transected with a linear stapler. An hand sewn side-to-side anastomosis is performed extracorporeally. In very simple cases, the ileocolic vascular pedicle is transected first with a 30-mm vascular stapler; transection and formation of the ileo-colic anastomosis are then performed intracorporeally. Mobilization of ascending colon is required if neoplasm is located in terminal ileum.

9.3 Surgical techniques for the treatment of adhesions

The patient should be secured with a bean bag, and a modified lithotomy position should be considered for posssible intraoperative endoscopy. Two monitors are ideal for this surgery. The site of first trocar placement should be carefully planned away from existing scars. The 30° scope provides excellent visualization. The pneumoperitoneum should never exceed 15 mmHg. The bowel should be examined for perforation and signs of ischemia. Free fluid should be aspirated and sent for gram staining, amylase, bilirubin, and culture. To facilitate exposure, table tilt, and external manual compression of the abdominal wall can be used. Second and third ports can be added to avoid excessive tenting of the abdominal wall. One of the most dreaded complications in laparoscopic management of small bowel obstruction is enterotomy. In a single comparative study (Wullstein & Gross, 2003), the risk of perforation was 27% in the laparoscopic group which was clearly higher than in the open group. The real concern, however, is that the bowel injury may be missed at the time of operation, with potential devastating consequences. The risk of bowel injury can be diminished by following good surgical technique. Bowel graspers with non-locking handles should be used gently to run the bowel. Exposure can be achieved by pushing with closed instruments rather than by grasping. The small bowel should be inspected in a retrograde fashion beginning from the caecum and decompressed bowel until the point of transition is identified. Energy-based devices should be avoided to divide adhesions. There should be a low threshold for conversion and it is not to be considered as a sign of failure but just a good clinical judgement. Conversion is not correlated to the number of previous surgeries (Navez et al., 1998). However, it may be predicted by bowel distension over 4 cm, a documented history of dense adhesions, and the presence of complete distal obstruction (Navez et al., 1998).

10. Conclusions

Small bowel diseases are rare and difficult to identify because diagnosis is late and often made on the base of the evidence of their complications. Small bowel laparoscopic surgery is extremely challenging, due to technical difficulties during mobilization of the intestinal loops, especially if dilated as a consequence of an occlusion. Nevertheless, after an adequate learning curve and with the help of small bowel endoscopic diagnostic tools, laparoscopic surgery of the small bowel can be considered as a feasible, safe and extremely accurate diagnostic and therapeutic choice for several small bowel diseases.

11. References

Abbas MA., Al-Kandari M. & Dashti FM. (2001). Laparoscopic-assisted resection of bleeding jejunal leiomyoma. *Surg Endosc*, 15, 1359-1362.

Albaz O., Iroatulam AJN., Nessim A., Weiss EG., Nogueras JJ. & Wexer SD. (2000). Comparision of laparoscopic assisted and conventional ileo-colic resection for Crohn's disease. *Eur J Surg*, 166, 213–217.

Ballantyne GH. (2002). The pitfalls of laparoscopic surgery: challenges for robotics and telerobotic surgery. *Surg Laparosc Endosc Percutan Tech*, 12, 1–5.

Berguer R. (1998). Surgical technology and the ergonomics of laparoscopic instruments. *Surg Endosc*, 12, 458–62

Bilimoria KY., Bentrem DJ. & Wayne JD. (2009). Small bowel cancer in United States. *Ann Surg*, 249, 63-71

Blay JY.; Bonvalot S. & Casali P. (2005). GIST consensus meeting panelists. Consensus meeting for the management of gastrointestinal stromal tumors. Report of the GIST Consensus Conference of 20–21 March 2004, under the auspices of ESMO. *Ann Oncol*, 16, 566–578

Bobby VMD., McKay D. & Gardiner K. (2011). Laparoscopic versus Open surgery for small bowel Crohn's disease. *Cochrane Database of Systematic Reviews*, 1, CD006956

Bodner J.; Chemelli A.; Zelger B. & Kafka R. (2005). Bleeding Meckel's diverticulum. *J Am Coll Surg*, 200: 631

Carrasco Rojas (2004). Minimally invasive surgery of small intestine. *Rev Gastroenterol Mex*, 69, Suppl1, 51-7

Carter MJ., Lobo AJ. & Travis SPL. (2004). Guidelines for the management of inflammatory bowel disease in adults. *Gut*, 53, 1-16.

Coco C, Rizzo G, Manno A, Mattana C & Verbo A. (2010). Surgical treatment of small bowel neoplasms. *Eur Rev Med Pharmacol Sci.*, 14, 327-33.

Crump M., Gospodarowicz M. & Shepherd FA. (1999). Lymphoma of the gastrointestinal tract. *Semin Oncol*, 26, 324-7

Cullen JJ., Kelly KA., Moir CR., Hodge DO., Zinsmeister AR. & Melton LJ 3rd. Surgical management of Meckel's diverticulum. An epidemiologic, population-based study. *Ann Surg*, 220, 564-568; discussion 568-569

Demetri GD., Benjamin R. & Blanke CD. (2004). Optimal management of patients with gastrointestinal stromal tumors. Expansion and update of NCCN Clinical Practice Guidelines. *J Natl Compr Care Netw*, 2, 51-526

Duepree H-J., Senagore AJ., Delaney CP., Brady KM. & Fazio VW. (2002). Advantages of laparoscopic resection for ileocecal Crohn's disease. *Dis Colon Rectum*, 45, 605–610.

Duh QY. (1998). Small bowel obstruction. *Endosurgery*. Churchill Livingstone, New York, 425–431

Dunker MS., Stiggelbout AM., Van Hogezand RA., Ringers J., Griffioen G. & Bemelman WA. (1998). Quality of life, cosmesis and body image after laparoscopic-assisted and open ileocolic resection for Crohn's disease. *Surg Endosc*, 12, 1334-40.

Ehrmantraut W. & Sardi A. (1997). Laparoscopy-assisted small bowel resection. *Am Surg*, 996-1001

Ell C, Remke S, May A, Helou L, Henrich R. & Mayer G (2002). The first prospective controlled trial comparing wireless capsule endoscopy with push enteroscopy in chronic gastrointestinal bleeding. *Endoscopy*, 34, 685-689

Eshuis EJ, Slors JFM, Stokkers PCF, Sprangers MAG, Ubbink DT, Cuesta MA, Pierik EGJM. & Bemelman WA. (2010). Long-term outcomes following laparoscopically assisted versus open ileo-colic resection for Crohn's disease. *BJS*, 97, 563–568.

Everett M. & Gutman H. (2008). Surgical management of gastrointestinal stromal tumors: analysis of outcome with respect to surgical margins and technique. *J Surg Oncol*, 98, 588-93

Fevang B-TS, Fevang J & Lie SA. (2004). Long-term prognosis after operation for adhesive small bowel obstruction. *Ann Surg*, 240, 193–201

Foster NM., McGory ML., Zingmond DS. & Ko CY. (2006). Small bowel obstruction: a population-based appraisal. *J Am Coll Surg*, 203, 170–176

Gerson LB. (2009). Capsule endoscopy and deep enteroscopy: indications for the practicing clinician. *Gastroenterology*, 137, 1197-201

Ghosheh B. & Salameh JR. (2007). Laparoscopic approach to acute small bowel obstruction: review of 1061 cases. *Surg Endosc*, 21, 1945–1949

Gill SS., Heuman DM. & Mihas A.(2001). Small intestinal neoplasm. *J Clin Gastroenterol*, 33, 267-82

Hartmann D, Schmidt H, Bolz G, Schilling D, Kinzel F, Eick-hoff A, Huschner W, Moller K, Jakobs R, Reitzig P, Weickert U, Gellert K, Schultz H, Guenther K, Hollerbuhl H, Schoenleben K, Schulz HJ. & Riemann JF. (2005). A prospective two-center study comparing wireless capsule endoscopy with intraoperative enteroscopy in patients with obscure GI bleeding. *Gastrointest Endosc*, 61, 826-832

Hasson H. (1974). Open laparoscopy: a report of 150 cases. *J Reprod Med*, 12, 234–238

Heinicke JM., Tedaldi R. & Muller C. (1997). An unusual manifestation of Meckel's diverticulum: bleeding and perforation — a case report. *Swiss Surg*, 3, 97–9

Higaki S., Saito Y. & Akazawa A. (2001). Bleeding Meckel's diverticulum in an adult. *Hepatogastroenterology*, 48, 1628-30

Howe JR., Karnell LH., Menck HR. & Scott-Conner C. (1999). The American College of Surgeons Commission on Cancer and the American Cancer Society. Adenocarcinoma of the small bowel: review of the National Cancer Data Base, 1985-1995. *Cancer*, 86, 2693-706

Hutchins RR., Bani Hani A., Kojodjojo P., Ho R. & Snooks SJ. (2001) Adenocarcinoma of the small bowel. *ANZ J Surg*, 71, 428-37

Jones BH., Fleischer DE., Sharma VK., Heigh RI., Shiff AD., Hernandez JL. & Leighton JA. (2005) Yield of repeat wireless video capsule endoscopy in patients with obscure gastrointestinal bleeding. *Am J Gastroenterol*, 100, 1058-1064

Kelling G. (1901). Die Tamponade der Speiseroehre und des magens mit beigsamen instrumenten. Verdhandlungen der Gesellschaft Deutscher Naturtorscher und Aerzte. *Vogel verlag Leipzig*, 73, 117–119

Keuchel M. & Hagenmuller F. (2005). Small bowel endoscopy. *Endoscopy*, 37, 122-132

Kok KY., Mathew VV. & Yapp SK (1998). Laparoscopic-assisted small bowel resection for a bleeding leiomyoma. *Surg Endosc*, 12, 995-996

Kong MS., Chen CY., Tzen KY., Huang MJ., Wang KL. & Lin JN. (1993). Technetium-99m pertechnetate scan for ectopic gastric mucosa in children with gastrointestinal bleeding. *J Formos Med Assoc*, 92, 717–20

Kulke MH. & Meyer RJ. (1999). Carcinoid tumors. *N Engl J Med*, 340, 858–68

Kumar R., Tripathi M., Chandrashekar N. Agarwala S, Kumar A, Dasan JB & Malhotra A. (2005). Diagnosis of ectopic gastric mucosa using 99Tcm-pertechnetate: spectrum of scintigraphic findings. *Br J Radiol*; 78:714-20

Lee KH., Yeung CK., Tam YH., Ng WT. & Yip KF. (2000). Laparascopy for definitive diagnosis and treatment of gastrointestinal bleeding of obscure origin in children. *J Pediatr Surg*, 35, 1291-1293

Leijonmarck CE., Bonman-Sandelin K., Frisell J. & Raf L. (1986). Meckel's diverticulum in the adult. *Br J Surg*, 73, 146-149

Lepage C., Bouvier AM., Manfredi S. Dancourt V. & Faivre J. (2006). Incidence and management of primary malignant small bowel cancer: a well-defined French population study. *Am J Gastroenterol*, 101, 2826-32

Lewis BS. & Swain P. (2002). Capsule endoscopy in the evaluation of patients with suspected small intestinal bleeding: Results of a pilot study. *Gastrointest Endosc*, 56, 349-353

Lin S., Suhocki PV., Ludwig KA. & Shetzline MA. (2002). Gastrointestinal bleeding in adult patients with Meckel's diverticulum: the role of technetium 99m pertechnetate scan. *South Med J*, 95, 1338–41

Litynski GS. (1998). Erich Muhe and the rejection of laparoscopic cholecystectomy: a surgeon ahead of his time. *J Soc Laparosc Surg*, 2, 341–346

Loh DL. & Munro FD. (2003). The role of laparoscopy in the management of lower gastrointestinal bleeding. *Pediatr Surg Int*, 19, 266-267

Lowney JK., Deitz DW., Birnbaum EH., Kodner IJ., Mutch MG. & Fleshman JW. (2005). Is there any difference in recurrence rates in laparoscopic ileo-colic resection for Crohn's disease compared with conventional surgery? *Dis Colon Rectum*, 49, 58–63.

Maartense S., Dunker MS., Slors JFM., Cuesta MA., Pierik EGJM., Gouma DJ., Hommes DW., Sprangers MA. & Bemelman WA. (2006). Laparoscopic-Assisted Versus Open ileo-colic Resection for Crohn's Disease. *Ann Surg*, 243, 143–149.

Mak SY., Roach SC. & Sukumar SA. (2006). Small bowel obstruction: computed tomography features and pitfalls. *Curr Probl Diagn Radiol*, 35, 65–74

Martinez-Ares D., Gonzalez-Conde B., Yanez J., Estevez E., Arnal F, Lorenzo J., Diz-Lois MT. & Vazquez-Iglesias JL. (2004). Jejunal leiomyosarcoma, a rare cause of obscure gastrointestinal bleeding diagnosed by wireless capsule endoscopy. *Surg Endosc*, 18, 554-556

Miller G., Boman J., Shrier I. & Gordon PH. (2000). Etiology of SBO. *Am J Surg*, 180, 33–36

Miller G., Boman J., Shrier I. & Gordon PH. (2000). Natural history of patients with adhesive small bowel obstruction. *Br J Surg*, 87, 1240–1247

Milsom JW., Hammerhofer KA., Bohm B., Marcello P., Elson P. & Fazio VW. (2001). Prospective randomised trial comparing laparoscopic vs conventional surgery for refractory ileocolic Crohn's disease. *Dis Colon Rectum*, 44, 1–9.

Milsom JW., Lavery IC., Bohm B. & Fazio VW. (1993). Laparoscopically assisted ileocolectomy in Crohn's disease. *Surg Laparosc Endosc*, 3, 77–80.

Morgan DR., Mylankal K, Barghouti N. & Dixon MF. (2000). Small bowel haemangioma with local lymph node involvement presenting as intussusception. *J Clin Pathol*, 53, 552-3

Munkholm P. & Binder V. (2004). *Clinical features and natural history of Crohn's disease. Kirsner's inflammatory bowel diseases.* 6th Edition; 289–300.

Navez B., Arimont JM & Guiot P. (1998) Laparoscopic approach in acute small bowel obstruction. A review of 68 patients. *Hepatogastroenterology*, 45, 2146–2150

Nelson H., Sargent DJ. & Wieand HS. (2004). A comparison of laparoscopically assisted and open colectomy for colon cancer. *N Engl J Med*, 350, 2050-9

Neugut AI., Jacobson JS., Suh S. Mukherjee R. & Arber N. (1998). The epidemiology of cancer of the small bowel. Cancer *Epidemiol Biomarkers Prev*, 7, 243–51

Neugut AI., Marvin MR., Rella VA. & Chabot JA. (1997). An overview of adenocarcinoma of the small intestine. *Oncology*, 11, 529

Nguyen NQ., Rayner CK. & Schoeman MN. (2005). Push enteroscopy alters management in a majority of patients with obscure gastrointestinal bleeding. *J Gastrointestinal Hepatol*, 20, 716-721

North JH. & Pack MS. (2000). Malignant tumors of the small intestine: a review of 114 cases. *Am Surg*, 66, 46–51

Novitsky YW., Kercher KW., Sing RF. & Heniford BT. (2006). Long-term outcomes of laparoscopic resection of gastric gastrointestinal stromal tumors. *Ann Surg*, 243, 738–745

Park JJ., Wolff BG., Tollefson MK., Walsh EE. & Larson DR. Meckel diverticulum: the Mayo Clinic experience with 1476 patients. Ann Surg; 241: 529-533

Puligandla PS., Becker L., Driman D., Prokopiw I., Taves D. & Davies ET. (2001). Inverted Meckel's diverticulum presenting as chronic anemia: case report and literature review. *Can J Surg*, 44, 458–9

Reissman P., Salky BA., Pfeifer J., Edye M., Jagelman DG. & Wexner SD. (1996). Laparoscopic surgery in the management of inflammatory bowel disease. *Am J Surg*, 171, 47–51.

Rerksuppaphol S., Hutson JM. & Oliver MR. (2004). Ranitidine-enhanced 99mtechnetium pertechnetate imaging in children improves the sensitivity of identifying heterotopic gastric mucosa in Meckel's diverticulum. *Pediatr. Surg Int*, 20, 323-325

Reissman P., Teoh TA. & Skinner K. (1996). Adhesion formation after laparoscopic anterior resection in a porcine model: a pilot study. *Surg Laparosc Endosc*, 6, 136–139

Rivas H., Cacchione RN. & Allen JW. (2003). Laparoscopic management of Meckel's diverticulum in adults. *Surg Endosc*, 17, 620-622

Robinson TN. & Stiegmann GV. (2004). Minimally invasive surgery. *Endocopy*, 36, 48–51

Ruh J., Paul A., Dirsch O., Kaun M. & Broelsch CE. (2010) Laparoscopic resection of perforated Meckel's diverticulum in a patient with clinical symptoms of acute appendicitis. *Surg Endosc*, 4207-14.

Sanders LE. (1995). Laparoscopic treatment of Meckel's diverticulum. Obstruction and bleeding managed with minimal morbidity. *Surg Endosc*, 9, 724-727

Sass DA., Chopra KB., Finkelstein SD. & Schauer PR. (2004). Jejunal gastrointestinal stromal tumor: a cause of obscure gastrointestinal bleeding. *Arch Pathol Lab Med*, 128, 214-217

Seror D., Feigin E., Szold A., Allweis TM., Carmon M., Nissan S. & Freund HR. (1993). How conservatively can postoperative small bowel obstruction be treated? *Am J Surg*, 165, 121-125

Shalaby RY., Soliman SM., Fawy M. & Samaha A. (2005). Laparoscopic management of Meckel's diverticulum in children. *J Pediatr Surg*, 40, 62-7

Shebani KO., Souba WW., Finkelstein DM., Stark PC., Elgadi KM., Tanabe KK. & Ott MJ. (1999). Prognosis and survival in patients with gastrointestinal tract carcinoid tumors. *Annals of Surgery*, 229, 815-823

Soltero MJ. & Bill AH. (1976). The natural history of Meckel's Diverticulum and its relation to incidental removal. A study of 202 cases of diseased Meckel's Diverticulum found in King County, Washington, over a fifteen year period. *Am J Surg*, 132, 168-173

Strickland P., Lourie DJ., Suddleson EA., Blitz JB. & Stain SC. (1999). Is laparoscopy safe and effective treatment of acute small bowel obstruction? *Surg Endosc*, 13, 695-698

Sutton R., Doran HE., Williams EM., Vora J., Vinjamuri S., Evans J., Campbell F., Raraty MG., Ghaneh P., Hartley M., Poston GJ. & Neoptolemos JP. (2003). Surgery for midgut carcinoid. *Endocrine-Related Cancer*, 10, 469-81

Tan YM. & Zheng ZX. (2005). Recurrent torsion of a giant Meckel's diverticulum. *Dig Dis Sci*, 50, 1285-7

Thoreson R. & Cullen JJ. (2007). Pathophysiology of Inflammatory Bowel disease: An overview. *Surg Clin N Am*, 87, 575-585.

Travis SP., Stange EF., Lémann M., Oresland T., Chowers Y., Forbes A., D'Haens G., Kitis G., Cortot A., Prantera C., Marteau P., Colombel JF., Gionchetti P., Bouhnik Y., Tiret E., Kroesen J., Starlinger M. & Mortensen NJ. (2006). European Crohn's and Colitis Organisation. European evidence based consensus on the diagnosis and management of Crohn's disease: current management. *Gut*, 55 (Suppl 1), i16-35.

Uchikoshi F., Ito T., Nezu R., Tanemura M., Kai Y., Mizushima T., Nakajima K., Tamagawa H., Matsuda C. & Matsuda (2004). H. Advantages of laparoscopic-assisted surgery for recurrent Crohn disease. *Surg Endosc*, 18, 1675-1679.

Veress J. (1938). Neues Instrument Zur Ausfuhrung von brustoder Bachpunktionen und Pneumothoraybehundlung. *Deutsch Med Wochenschr*, 64, 1480-148

Warneke RM., Walser E., Faruqi S., Jafri S., Bhutani MS. & Raju GS. (2004). Cap-assisted endoclip placement for recurrent ulcer hemorrhage after repeatedly unsuccessful endoscopic treatment and angiographic embolization: case report. *Gastrointest Endosc*, 60, 309-312

Witteman BJ., Janssens AR., Griffioen G. & Lamers CB. (1993). Villous tumours of the duodenum. An analysis of the literature with emphasis on malignant transformation. *Neth J Med*, 42, 5-11

Wong JH., Suhaili DN. & Kok KY. (2005). Fish bone perforation of Meckel's diverticulum: a rare event? *Asian J Surg*, 28, 295–6

Wullstein C. & Gross E. (2003). Laparoscopic compared with conventional treatment of acute adhesive small bowel obstruction. *Br J Surg*, 90, 1147–1151

Yamaguchi T. & Yoshikawa K. (2003), Enhanced CT for initial localization of active lower gastrointestinal bleeding. *Abdom Imaging*, 28, 634-636

Yao KA., Talamonti MS., Nemcek A., Angelos P., Chrisman H., Skarda J., Benson AB., Rao S. & Joehl RJ. (2001). Indications and results of liver resection and hepatic chemoembolization for metastatic gastrointestinal neuroendocrine tumors. *Surgery*, 130, 677–685

Zani A., Eaton S., Rees CM. & Pierro A. (2008). Incidentally detected Meckel diverticulum: to resect or not to resect? *Ann Surg*, 247, 276-281

Part 2

Urogynecological Endoscopy

5

Urology: The Home of Endoscopy

Rastislav Hejj, Marie McNulty and John G. Calleary

Department of Urology,
North Manchester General Hospital,
Pennine Acute Hospitals NHS Trust
Crumpsall, Manchester M8 5RB
United Kingdom

1. Introduction

1.1 Place of endoscopy in urology

Urology is truly the home of endoscopy. Starting with the introduction of first cystoscope, Urology has been at the forefront of endoscopic use in clinical practice. Endoscopy is used in both diagnosis and therapeutic settings (Table 1). Currently, endoscopy is used for diagnosis of bladder pathology and this is primarily with the use of flexible instruments under local anaesthesia. It is the gold standard for the identification of urethral stricture disease and diagnostic standard for the identification of intravesical *Transitional Cell Carcinoma (TCC)* and the primary follow-up tool for non-muscle invasive TCC. Transurethral Resection of Bladder Tumour (TURBT) is the mainstay for pathological diagnosis of Transitional Cell Carcinoma (TCC). Its efficacy has been improved by modern technical developments such as blue-light cystoscopy. This staging provides information on whether more radical therapies are necessary or whether continued endoscopic surveillance can be continued.

Relief of ureteric obstruction often involves stenting of the relevant ureter. Above the bladder, rigid endoscopy is used diagnose ureteric stone disease. Treatment of identified stones is usually endoscopic, using either Holmium laser or lithoclast technology. In recent times this practice seemed to have shifted toward a greater role for Shock wave lithotripsy.

In the sphere of organ ablative surgery, since the introduction of laparoscopy to Urology it has been possible to apply endourological techniques to ablative procedures. Thus laparoscopic nephrectomy is now the standard for radiological T1-T2 lesions where partial ablation is inappropriate. This chapter proposes to track the use of endoscopy in Urology and to show why Endoscopy and Endoscopic techniques have become central to Urological diagnosis and treatment.

1.2 History of endoscopy in urology

This section is not meant to be the didactic history of Urological Endoscopy. For that we would suggest Mr J Shah's review (Shah 2002) or Dr Herr's review in the Journal of Endourology (Herr 2006). Rather it is an attempt to provide an insight into developments and timelines in the evolution of Urological endoscopy.

Organ	Endoscopy used for Diagnosis D/ Therapy T/ Both B	Open or Endoscopic Techniques as the prime Surgical modality	Conditions (examples)
Urethra	B	E >> O	Stricture, HUA, Pain, Foreign bodies, Malignancy
Prostate / Bladder neck Benign Malignancy	B T	E >>> O O = E	Obstruction, Malignancy,
Bladder Benign Malignancy	B but D >>T B	E >>> O E > O	Strorage symptoms, HUA, Malignancy, Foreign bodies
Ureter including renal collecting system Benign Malignant	B B but T >> D	E >>> O O = E	Urolithiasis, HUA, Malignancy, Stricture, Functional obstruction eg Pelvi-ureteric-junction
Kidney Benign Malignant	Little place T	E = O	Glomerulonephritis Renal Cell malignancy

Table 1. The place of Endoscopic Urological procedures in the treatment of Urological disease

The first to attempt to visualise the urogenital tract was by Bozzini in 1806. His "Lichtleiter" consisted of a funnel, candle and a reflector. Its problem was of poor illumination so much so that from the practical viewpoint it was unusable. Further improvements made by Ségales and Fischer led to the development by Desormeaux of a cystoscope where illumination was provided by an alcohol and turpentine lamp. This was the first instrument to be used for a therapeutic manoeuvre. Desormeaux, has been called "the Father of Cystoscopy", in part because he was one of the first to introduce a Lichleiter into a patient. Cruise, Newman and especially Nitze were responsible for modifications which improved illumination including the use of intra-corporeal bulbs. In 1887 Nitze introduced a cystoscope which did not require a cooling apparatus and through which biopsies could be taken.

In 1889 Boisseau du Rocher introduced a twin sheath modification which allowed simultaneous visualisation and instrumentation/ irrigation. Albarran in 1896 introduced a catheter deflector. Further developments in both the USA and Europe in illumination allowed the use of prisms as lenses. These developments led to the resectoscope which was first introduced in 1926 by Stern and modified by McCarthy in 1931 to produce the Stern-McCarthy resectoscope. This was the first instrument recognisable as a modern resectoscope. Trans-Urethral Resection of the Prostate / Bladder lesions was made possible through the work of Hertz and DeForest who described the use of high frequency current for and vacuum tube that made tissue resection possible. Their work was further progressed by Wappler and Wyeth (cutting current) and W.T. Bovie and G.H. Leibel (coagulating current). The true modern resection instrument was then developed by Frederick Wappler in 1931 and resection of the prostate (TURP) was first described in a published account by Nesbitt in 1943.

Flexible instruments were initially developed by Mikulicz in 1881 who attached a 30 degree deflection mechanism to a cystoscope and performed an oesohagoscopy. The first semi-flexible cystoscopy was performed using a Wolf and Schindler instrument in 1936. Ureteroscopy was first performed in the early 1900`s using a Brandford Lewis instrument.

As alluded to above, the earliest instruments used external combustible light sources. Their main disadvantage was of poor illumination and a certain danger of burns to their operator and the patient. Candles gave way to alcohol burners which produced more light but the heat they produced required the addition of a cooling device. The field of view was still limited to the diameter of the instrument although the light intensity was increased.

The major improvement came from Edison`s invention of the bulb in 1880. The development of the "Mignon" lamp allowed better illumination of the bladder from its position at the distal end of the cystoscope. Distal illumination remained the main stay until fibre-optics was applied to endoscope design in the 1950`s. Fibre-optics use the phenonomen of Multiple Total Internal Reflection. Professor Harold Hopkins and Narinder Kampany published in Nature in January 1954 on image transmission through unclad fibres. In the same edition Van Heel reports on image transmission through clad light fibres. Hence light could be transmitted through fibre-optic bundles and the target image viewed through the same telescope. To see a true image the fibres had to be coherenty arranged *i.e.* the fibres had to occupy the same relative position at either end. Hopkins also worked on rigid systems and the application of glass fibre innovations led to the rod-lens system currently used in most rigid endoscopes. The advantage of this system is the increased light intensity delivered to the target and the better image due to a reduction in light loss within the lens casing.

The development which will further revolutionise endoscopy is the development of distal sensors. These are based on either CCD (charge coupled device) or CMOS (complementary metal-oxide semi-conductor) technology. Both technologies register an image as an electrical charge proportional to the light intensity of the image. These charges / impulses are then processed and reformatted as a colour image. CCD cameras and telescopes are further along in development. Three chip (one for each of the prime colours) systems have resulted in increased visualisation and resolution. Its introduction has led to NBI (Narrow Band Imaging) technology which is discussed later. In a head to head comparison between fibre-optic and distal sensor endoscopes, Okhunov et al showed that distal sensor technology was superior in the 1000 procedures tested (Okhunov 2009).

2. Endoscopy of lower urinary tract

2.1 Flexible cystoscopy (figure 1)

Flexible cystoscopy permits direct visual inspection of the urethra and bladder following instillation of lubricant local anaesthetic gel. The instruments used currently predominantly use fibre-optic technology for light and image transmission. Hence they need a separate light source and usually a camera system. The indications are principally diagnostic (investigation of haematuria, the storage lower tract symptoms of frequency and urgency) where intravesical pathology is suspected and in the surveillance of patients with previously diagnosed and treated bladder cancer. The gradual introduction of newer technology such as distal sensor all digital endoscopes and narrow band imaging will improve resolution and thus detection of recurrent bladder TCC (Transitional Cell Carcinoma).

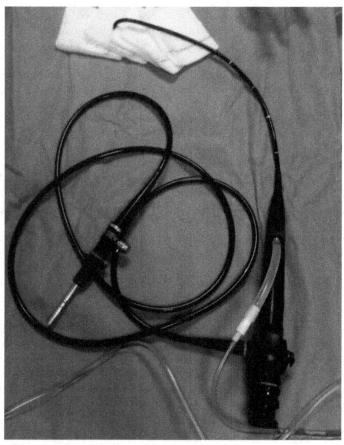

Fig. 1. Modern fibre-optic flexible cystoscope

In terms of therapeutic indications flexible cystoscopy can be used for biopsy and destruction of small tumours using diathermy fulguration or holmium laser vaporisation. Polymer based stents (eg JJ stents) inserted to relieve ureteric obstruction are usually removed at flexible cystoscopy and in some cases can even be inserted (Reynard et al., 2009). However the majority of such procedures are performed at rigid cystoscopy. Intravesical Botulinium-A toxin sub-mucosal injection performed through the flexible cystoscope is now a standard treatment for intractable storage symptoms resistant to oral anti-muscarinic agents . Complications of flexible cystoscopy include mild burning or bleeding on passing urine for a short period (common) and urinary tract infection requiring antibiotics (<5-10%- this rate can be reduced by prophylactic antibiotics).

2.2 Rigid Cystoscopy and Trans Urethral Resection of Bladder Tumour; TURBT
(Figure 2 shows instruments in common use)

Rigid cystoscopy as a diagnostic tool has been virtually replaced by flexible cystoscopy. However it is the main vehicle through which reasonable bladder biopsies are taken and a pre-request to many endoscopic procedures. Instruments are available for paediatric and adults and the adult instruments usually are 18-22 Ch in diameter.

TURBT is the most important diagnostic procedure for bladder tumours as the histological evaluation of the resected tissue allows a clinician to distinguish between non-muscle invasive ("superficial") and muscle invasive bladder cancer. The most common histological sub-type of bladder cancer is Transitional Cell Carcinoma (TCC). 75-85% of newly diagnosed bladder TCC are non-muscle invasive ("superficial") and for these TURBT is also the definitive treatment. The remaining 15-25% are muscle invasive, requiring radical treatment (either surgical- radical cystectomy, or radical radiotherapy).

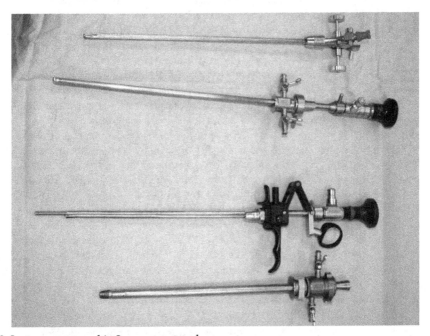

Fig. 2. Instruments used in Lower tract endoscopy
From top to bottom; Modern Albarran catheterizing bridge, Rigid cystoscope in its 22f sheath, Resectoscope working element with its lens and resectoscope sheath and obturator.

TURBT starts with bimanual palpation to assess whether a tumour mass is palpable and to ascertain whether its mobile. A fixed mass implies a more locally advanced disease process. Following this, a rigid cystoscopy is performed to visualise the bladder tumour and assess the size (in cm), appearance (?papillary, ?solid, ?flat/red area) , position (base, lateral wall, posterior wall, dome) and their relationship to the ureteric orifici.

A resectoscope is then placed per-urethrally with an external diameter 18Ch and 28 Ch. Identified lesions are then resected using a loop electrode and sent for histology. Bladder muscle (muscularis propria) should be present in resected tissue as the presence of TCC in muscle is the hallmark of muscle invasive disease. The resected tissue is then removed using an Ellik evacuator and diathermy to bleeding points performed with a rollerball electrode. At the end of the procedure, repeat bimanual palpation is performed as a means of ensuring complete resection of the lesion. A 3-way irrigation catheter is inserted and removed within 24-48 hours unless an extra-peritoneal perforation has occurred. For tumours which appear superficial, Intravesical Mitomycin C within 24 hours of resection has been shown to reduce number of recurrences by 39% (Sylvester et al., 2004). Currently the only place for open procedures in TCC diagnosis and management is in radical cystectomy and a urinary diversion procedure. However, the technique of laparoscopic cystectomy has been developed (Parra 1992) and is gaining acceptance.

2.3 Trans-Urethral Resection of Prostate (TURP)

While the majority of men are managed medically, TURP is the gold standard surgical treatment for lower urinary tract symptoms (LUTS) due to benign prostatic hyperplasia (BPH) causing bladder outlet obstruction (BOO). TURP involves resection of prostatic adenomatous tissue to the level of the prostatic capsule. Prostatic chippings are flushed into the bladder during resection by irrigation fluid (usually 1,5% glycine) and at the end of the procedure washed out from the bladder (using Ellik bladder evacuator) and sent for histological examination. The most important landmarks are the ureteric orificii proximally and the Veru montanum distally. The Veru is the marker of the proximal limit of the external sphincter, damage to which results in stress urinary incontinence.

TURP is performed for men with voiding symptoms which fail to respond to medical treatment (alpha-blockers, 5-alpha reductase inhibitors), for men with urinary retention (failed trial of catheter removal on medical treatment) and for those who develop complications of bladder outlet obstruction especially renal impairment. Complications are as follows severe bleeding requiring blood transfusion (1-2%), sepsis (3%), TUR syndrome (<1%), urinary incontinence (<1%), bladder neck stenosis/ urethral stricture (3-5%), retrograde ejaculation (80-100%) and erectile dysfunction (approximately 10%). Alternative surgical treatments include "Greenlight" laser ablation or Holmium laser enucleation, both of which are performed under cystoscopic guidance. Smaller prostates are also managed endoscopicaly using a Bladder Neck Incision (BNI). Open surgery for benign prostatic disease is now extremely rare and performed only when the prostate is > 100 gr or if there is a concurrent bladder stone (McAllister 2010).

2.4 Technological advances in the endoscopic diagnosis of bladder cancer

The development of distal sensor technologies has led to development of techniques which aim to increase the diagnostic capability of white-light cystoscopy (WLC) in the detection of TCC. Probably the two landmark developments are Photodynamic diagnosis (PDD), also referred to as "fluorescence cystoscopy" and Narrow-Band Imaging (NBI).

2.4.1 Photodynamic diagnosis (PDD)

PDD requires the intravesical instillation of a fluorescent agent (e.g. 5-aminolaevulinic acid (5-ALA), or its ester hexaminolevulinate) before performing blue-light cystoscopy. The principle of PDD is based on the difference in uptake of fluorescence molecules in normal and pathologic tissue. Absorption of light of an appropriate wavelength causes excitation of the fluorophore molecule which on returning to its ground state emits a photon equivalent to the energy difference between these states. Endoscopes with specially developed light sources and filters are used, and with the aid of a foot pedal or push-button on the camera one can easily switch from WLC to PDD. By illuminating the bladder wall with blue light, the malignant tissue appears intensely pink or red on a blue background (Cauberg et al., 2009). Clinical trials have shown that the detection of TCC with PDD is superior to WLC with reported sensitivities of 82-97% for PDD versus 62-84% for WLC. With regard to the detection of CIS lesions, PDD performs significantly better than WLC with detection rates of 92-97% versus 56-68%, respectively. PDD use may also have an impact on recurrence rate. This has been studied by cystoscopic re-evaluation six weeks following initial resection using WLC or Blue light cystoscopy. Results of published studies seem to show a statistically significant reduction in residual tumour if resection was performed with PDD (25-53% for white-light resection vs 4-32% for PDD-assisted resection). However, PDD has a relatively low specificity, ranging from 41 to 98% and false-positive fluorescence can be induced by inflammation, scarring after TUR, prior intravesical therapy and tangential illumination of mucosa (Cauberg et al., 2009). It is hoped that the initial cost of the technology will be recouped by an increased recurrence-free survival or progression-free survival. This remains to be proven in larger randomised clinical trials.

2.4.2 Narrow-band imaging (NBI)

NBI is an optical image enhancement technique designed to enhance the contrast between mucosal surfaces and microvascular structures without the use of dyes. It is based on the phenomenon that the depth of light penetration into the mucosa increases with increasing wavelength. The tissue surface is illuminated with light of a narrow bandwidth, with centre wavelengths in the blue (415 nm) and green (540 nm) spectrum of light. Since these specific wavelengths are strongly absorbed by haemoglobin, the vascular structures appear dark brown or green against a pink or white mucosal background. Systems that have integrated NBI and WLC are commercially available. With the push of a button, the NBI mode is activated by mechanical insertion of the narrow-band filter in front of the white-light source. NBI has not been as extensively investigated as PDD and therefore it is hard to know the effect of inflammation, previous intra-vesical instillations or scarring on its sensitivity (Cauberg et al., 2009). The inherent advantage of NBI over PDD is that it avoids the physical discomfort and extra cost associated with requirement for instillation of the intra-vesical agent pre-operatively. The small number of studies performed comparing NBI to WLC suggested a non-significant improvement in the detection of bladder cancer, but more studies are needed to assess the benefit of NBI further.

2.5 Optical urethrotomy (figure 3)

Modern Urethral stricture diagnosis is primarily by flexible endoscopy. The initial endoscopy can identify the number of, diameter of and the rigidity of any identified strictures. Previously diagnosis was primarily by radiological means prompted by clinical suspicion. It is possible to definitively treat a stricture by endoscopic means by performing a Direct Visual Internal Urethrotomy, using an optical urethrotome.

An Optical urethrotome has a straight (0 degree) lens, cold knife and a channel for the introduction of a guide-wire into the bladder. This guidewire allows a urethral catheter to be passed if bleeding obscures visualisation of the lumen. A cold-knife incision is made at the 12 o'clock position until the lumen of the strictured segment is approximately the same as of the remaining urethra. A 16-18 Fr catheter is inserted post-operatively and removed after 2-5 days. Optical urethrotomy is most suitable for strictures less than 1 cm in length, of the Bulbar urethra (71% success rate) and for strictures with a calibre of greater than 15F (69% vs 36%). Recurrences, if they occur, will do so within 12 (56%) or 24 months (26%) months (Pansadoro 1996). For all other strictures the definitive treatment should still be open reconstructive surgery.

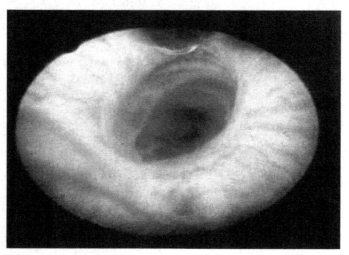

Fig. 3. Anterior Urethral stricture at Direct Visual Optical Urethrotomy (optical urethrotomy with a cold knife seen at 12 o`clock)

Endoscopy of upper urinary tract

2.6 Ureteroscopy (figure 4)

Ureteroscopy can be performed using semi-rigid or flexible instruments to allow visual inspection of ureter and renal pelvis (semi-rigid ureteroscope) and major and minor renal calyces (flexible ureteroscope). Semi-rigid ureteroscopes have high-density fibre-optic bundles for light (non-coherently arranged) and image transmission (coherently arranged to maintain image quality). The instrument can be bent by several degrees without the image being distorted, hence the description semi-rigid. The working tip of most current models is 7-8 Ch with the proximal end being 11-12 Ch. There is usually at least one working channel of at least 3 or 4 Ch (Reynard et al., 2009). In a flexible instrument, the operator can control the degree of deflection of the distal end (active deflection). Behind the actively deflecting tip is a segment of greater flexibility than the rest of the shaft. This section is able to undergo passive deflection (when the tip is fully actively deflected, by advancing the scope further, this flexible segment allows even more deflection). The fibre-optic bundles in flexible instruments are identical to those in semi-rigid scopes, only of smaller diameter. The price of the extra mobility is reduced image quality and light transmission (Reynard et al., 2009). The working tip of most current models is 7-8 Ch, with the proximal end of the scope 9-10 Ch. There is usually at least one working channel of at least 3.6 Ch. Flexible instruments are more expensive and less durable than semi-rigid scopes.

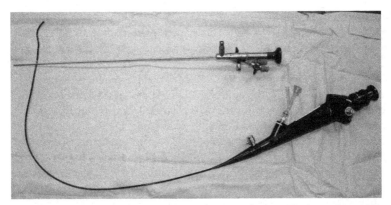

Fig. 4. Examples of Modern Upper Tract instruments in routine Urological use. Top: Semi-Rigid Ureteroscope. Bottom: Flexible Ureteroscope (fibre-optic technology)

The indications for ureteroscopy are either diagnostic (e.g. patient with haematuria and filling defect in upper urinary tract on contrast study) or therapeutic. The primary therapeutic use of Ureteroscopy is in upper tract stone disease (figure 5) where stone destruction can be achieved with laser, ultrasonic or EHL (electrohydrolic) technology. Fragments can be removed using a variety of baskets introduced through the working channel. Potential complications include stone migration (4%), ureteric injury (3.5%), sepsis (1%) and failure to reach stone (3.7%) (Geavlete 2006).

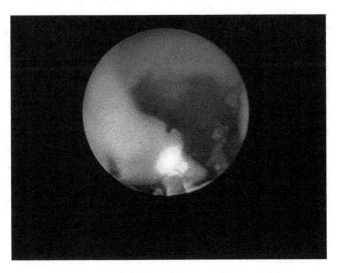

Fig. 5. Ureteroscopic holmium laser lithotripsy. Laser fibre at 6 o'clock with green aiming beam shining on the stone.

to the extent that, for stones requiring surgical treatment, open stone surgery is now the exception rather than the normal. The other main therapeutic indication is in selected cases of upper urinary tract transitional cell carcinoma (TCC).

2.7 Per-Cutaneous NephroLithotomy (PCNL)

The first PCNL was performed in 1976. Since then open nephrolithotomy has reduced in frequency to the current rate of < 1% of all stone procedures. The current treatment options are PCNL, Shock-wave lithotripsy and flexible ureteroscopy. PCNL is the 1st line treatment option for staghorn and other large renal stones (>2 cm in maximum diameter). A Staghorn stone is defined as a stone filling the entire renal pelvis and at least one (partial staghorn) or all of the calyces (complete staghorn). PCNL is also indicated for smaller stones in specific circumstances such as abnormal anatomy (e.g. horshoe kidney, calyceal diverticulum), failure of other treatment options (ureteroscopy, ESWL) or patient preference. PCNL is more invasive (higher morbidity) than ureteroscopy or ESWL but has a higher efficacy in single treatment stone clearance (especially for larger stones). Treatment of lower pole calyceal stones measuring 1-2 cm in maximum diameter remains a controversial issue. As stated above, the available options are flexible ureteroscopy, ESWL or PCNL. Access to the lower pole calyx by flexible ureteroscopy can be difficult and the stone-free rates after ESWL are lower than for stones in other parts of the kidney. This has led some to favour PCNL as the first line option for 1-2 cm stones in lower pole calyx. Two prospective, randomised studies tried to resolve this problem; Lower Pole Study I (Albala et al., 2001) and Lower Pole Study II (Pearle et al., 2005). Lower Pole Study I compared ESWL to PCNL for 1-3 cm stones localised in lower pole calyx. PCNL was more successful (95% vs 37%) but had higher morbidity. Lower Pole Study II compared ESWL to Ureteroscopy for <1 cm stones in lower pole calyx. Ureteroscopy was more successful in stone clearance (50% vs 35%) but due to relatively small number of patients (n=67) this result failed to achieve statistical significance. Despite these two studies the question of the best treatment for <2 cm lower pole calyceal stones remains difficult to answer and proper patient counselling about pros and cons of each therapeutic option is crucial.

How is PCNL performed? The patient has been traditionally placed prone, but over the recent years it has been demonstrated that PCNL is also feasible in supine position. Ureteric catheterisation (with or without balloon) is performed primarily to fill the collecting system which facilitates puncture (contrast and methylene blue injected through ureteric catheter dilates and opacifies collecting system) but also to minimise migration of stone fragments into the ureter. The puncture can be made under combined ultrasound and X-ray control or under fluoroscopy. Ultrasound makes it easier to identify, and therefore avoid damage to, neighbouring organs. In rare cases with complex anatomy, CT-guided renal access may be an option (Turk et al., 2010). The most common access is through the posterior lower pole calyx. It is the safest access point due to absence of major blood vessels (so called Brodel's avascular zone) and low risk of pleural injury. In selected cases (e.g.complex staghorn stones) a supra-costal upper pole access or even multiple punctures have been used. After successful puncture of the renal collecting system, dilatation of renal tract is performed-using Amplatz system, balloon or metallic dilators (choice depends on availability, experience and cost). After insertion of the nephroscope, the stone is disintegrated using ultrasound, laser, or pneumatic energy. Fragments are removed using suction (via ultrasound probe) or specially designed forceps. In complicated cases (or when second intervention is necessary), a self-retaining balloon nephrostomy tube tamponades the tract and maintains access to the collecting system. Although standard nephroscopes have shaft calibres of 24-30 F, "mini-perc" instruments are now available with shaft calibres of 12-20 F.

Mini-perc is the method of choice for PCNL in children (Turk et al., 2010). The value of mini-perc in adults hasn't been established (as treatment time increases with stone size and also with decreased instrument size- mini-perc in adults would be recommended only for <2 cm stones where many experts would argue that alternative options- ESWL or URS would be preferred). In uncomplicated cases, tubeless PCNL (with or without application of sealant or JJ stent) has been mentioned over the last few years as an alternative (Turk et al., 2010). The percutaneous route has also been used to treat PUJ (Pelvi-ureteric Junction) obstruction as a concurrent procedure to stone treatment.

The major complications of PCNL are infection, bleeding and internal organ injury. Many of the larger stones are either infection stones or cause obstruction. In view of this, peri-operative antibiotic prophylaxis is a standard of practice. The choice of antibiotic is guided by preoperative urine cultures and local antibiotic policies.

Bleeding following PCNL can be severe enough to require blood transfusion but rarely needs intervention such as embolisation or Nephrectomy. Internal organ injury can affect pleura (risk higher if attempting upper pole puncture), bowel (risk especially if bowel lies behind kidney- CT is therefore important to show the bowel position and plan the access) and rarely liver or spleen.

2.8 Relief of ureteric obstruction

Endoscopic placement of ureteric stents (ie Retrograde stent insertion) is the commonest method of relieving ureteric obstruction. Stents are either barium impregnated polymer compounds or metallic. Drainage occurs either through or around the tubes. The JJ shape contains coils at both ends to help retain the stent in its position. Retrograde stenting is used for both intrinsic and extrinsic malignant obstruction and less successfully for retroperitoneal obstruction due to fibrotic benign pathology. Prophylactic stenting is used prior to ESWL for large stones where the fragments could obstruct the ureter (ie Steinstrasse). Post-operatively stent placement is used to ensure urinary drainage following prolonged/ complicated ureteroscopy or PUJ procedures.

Retrograde stenting is performed usually under anaesthetic. The ureteric orifice is visualised at cystoscopy, it is then cannulated with an open-ended polymer catheter and retrograde studies are performed to outline the ureter and renal collecting system. A guide-wire is passed through the ureteric orifice into the collecting system (ideally upper pole calyx). The appropriate stent (dependent on patient height) is inserted over the guide-wire, under X-ray guidance, so that the upper end of the stent is in the correct position in renal collecting system. The guide-wire is then removed and both ends of stent subsequently coil (they have "memory").

The most common adult stents are 4.8-6 Fr and 22-28 cm long. Some stents have a hydrophilic coating (makes them more slippery and easier to insert), some are multi-length (no need to adjust according to patient's height). Endopyelotomy stents are wider towards the upper end (10-14 Fr)- to keep PUJ wide open while it heals.

The complications commonly associated with stent usage are storage LUTS (frequency, urgency) and haematuria. Stent migration is less common and can occur in both directions. Probably the biggest concern is stent calcification due to "forgotten stent". If only the lower end of the stent is calcified treatment can usually be completed endoscopically. Calcification of a stent above the bladder will require ureteroscopic lithotripsy, PCNL or even open surgery to facilitate removal.

3. Organ ablative surgery

While the majority of lower tract and stone surgical treatments are now performed endoscopically the field of organ ablation remains the domain of the "open" surgeon. However that is changing and started when the first laparoscopic trans-abdominal nephrectomy was performed in 1990 by Clayman and colleagues at Washington University. The progress of endoscopy techniques in organ ablative urological surgery is mirrored in the changed attitudes to laparoscopic nehrectomy and hence this procedure will be the focus of this section.

3.1 Laparoscopic nephrectomy

Following the initial nephrectomy, techniques have evolved so that laparoscopic radical nephrectomy is almost the standard procedure for T1- T2 tumours (those limited to the kidney and less than 7 cm *i.e.* T1 or less than 10 cm *i.e.* T2) where renal sparing procedures are inappropriate. In experienced hands T3 tumours (*i.e.* involving renal vein or vena cava) can also be removed using this endoscopic technique. The Oncological outcomes are almost identical with disease free survival rates of 94% and 95 % respectively for the open and laparoscopic approaches (Hemal 2007). When morbidity and return to normal function are analysed it appears that the laparoscopic approach to nephrectomy is better in all measured outcomes apart from a prolongation of operative time (Nandis 2008).

Indeed the debate around nephrectomy now centres on whether the NOTES approach to nephrectomy should be the method of choice. Preservation of renal tissue may be associated with an independent reduction in cardio-vascular and all causes mortality rates (Go 2004). This has led to the increased utilisation of partial nephrectomy for T1a (ie < 4 cm) lesions. While the open approach to partial nephrectomy is the more popular approach there are an increasing number of centres performing laparoscopic partial nephrectomy. For a more detailed description of laparoscopic techniques I would suggest Bishoff and Kavoussi`s Atlas of Laparoscopic Urologic Surgery (2007) as an introductory text.

Currently, in the field of organ ablative urology, laparoscopic techniques (including robotics) are commonly being used for nephrectomy, nephro-ureterectomy and radical prostatectomy. Their use in procedures such as retro-peritoneal lymph node dissection or radical cystectomy remains to be proven.

4. Conclusion

To the reader of this chapter, it may appear that we have only provided a summary of modern urology. Of itself this impression should illustrate clearly the central place of endoscopy and endoscopic techniques in modern urological practise. Obviously we could not describe all endoscopic techniques used in urology but we have tried to describe the more commonly performed procedures. In places we have shown how developments are further improving efficacy of endoscopic techniques and increasing the range of conditions treated by endoscopic means.

5. References

Albala, D.M.; Assimoss, D.G.; Clayman, R.V.; Densted, J.D.; Grasso, M. et al. (2001). Lower pole I: a prospective randomised trial of extracorporeal shock wave Lithotripsy and percutaneous nephrolithotomy for lower pole nephrolithiasis- Initial results. *J Urol*, 166, pp. 2072-2080

A. Alcaraz, L. Peri, A. Molina, I. Goicoechea, E. García, L. Izquierdo, M. Ribal. (2010) Feasibility of Transvaginal NOTES-Assisted Laparoscopic Nephrectomy. *European Urology*, Volume 57, Issue 2, Feb 2010. Pages 233-237 ISSN 0302 2838

Anger JT, Weinberg A, Suttorp MJ, Litwin MS and Shekelle PG. Outcomes of Intravesical Botulinum Toxin for Idiopathic Overactive Bladder Symptoms: A Systematic Review of the Literature. *J Urol* 2010; 183(6): pp 2258-2264.

Bishoff JT and Kavoussi LR (eds). (2007) *Atlas of Laparoscopic Urological Surgery*. 2007 Saunders, ISBN-13: 978-1-4160-2580-1, Philidelphia.

Cauberg, E.C.C.; De Bruin, D.M.; Faber, D.J.; Van Leeuwen, T.G.; De la Rosette,J.M.C.H; De Reijke, T.M.; (2009). A New Generation of Optical Diagnostics for Bladder Cancer: Technology, Diagnostic Accuracy, and Future Applications. *European Urology*, Vol. 56, Issue 2, August 2009, pp. 287-297, ISSN 0302 2838

Denstedt, J.; Khoury S. (2008). *Stone disease (2nd international consultation on stone disease)*, Editions 21, ISBN 0-9546956-7-4, Paris, France

Geavlete P, Georgescu D, Niţă G, Mirciulescu V, Cauni V. (2006) Complications of 2735 retrograde semi-rigid ureteroscopic procedures: a single centre experience. *J Endourol* 20, Mar 2006 , pp 179-185.

Go AS, Chertow GM, Fan D, McCulloch CE & Hsu CY. (2004) Chronic kidney disease and the risks of death, cardiovascular events and hospitalisation. *N Engl J Med* 351; (13): September 23 2004 pp 1296-1305.

Hemal AK, Kumar A, Kumar R, Wadhwa P, Seth A & Gupta NP. (2007) Laparoscopic versus open radical nephrectomy for large renal tumours: a longterm prospective comparison. *J Urol*; 177(3) March 2007: pp 862-866

Herr H. Early history of treatment of bladder tumours from Grunfeld`s polypenkneipe to the Stern-McCarthy resectoscope. (2006) *J Endourl* 2006; 20 (2); pp 85-91

McAllister WJ. Benign Prostatic Hyperplasia in Arya, M.; Shergill, I.S.; Kalsi J.S.; Muneer A.; Mundy A.R. (2010). *Viva Practice for the FRCS (Urol) Examination*, Radcliffe Publishing Ltd, ISBN-13: 978 184619 317 0, Oxon, United Kingdom

Nanidis TG, Antcliffe D, Kokkinos C, Borysiewicz CA, Darzi AW, Tekkis PP & Papalois VE. (2008) Laparoscopic versus open donor nephrectomy in renal transplantation: a meta-analysis. *Ann Surg* 247(1) January 2008; pp 58-70

Okhunov Z, Hruby GW, Mirabile G, Marruffo F, Lehman DS, Benson MC, Gupta M & Landman J. (2009). Prospective comparison of flexible fibreoptic and digital cystoscopies. *Urology* 2009; 74: 427-430

Pansadoro V and Emiliozzi P. (1996) Internal Urethrotomy in the management of anterior urethral strictures: long-term followup. *J Urol* 1996; 156(1):73-75

Parra RO, Andrus CH, Jones JP & Boullier JA. Laparoscopic cystectomy: Initial report on a new treatment for the retained bladder (1992). *J Urol* 148: pp 1140-1144

Pearle MS, Lingeman JE, Leveillee R, Kuo R, Preminger GM, Nadler RB, Macaluso J, Monga M, Kumar U, Dushinski J, Albala DM, Wolf JS Jr, Assimos D, Fabrizio M, Munch LC, Nakada SY, Auge B, Honey J, Ogan K, Pattaras J, McDougall EM, Averch TD, Turk T, Pietrow P, & Watkins S. (2005) Prospective, randomised trial comparing Shock wave lithotripsy and ureteroscopy for lower pole caliceal calculi 1cm or less. *J Urol* ; 173(6) june 2005, pp 2005-2009

Reynard, J.; Brewster, S.; Biers, S. (2009). *Oxford Handbook of Urology (2nd edition)*, Oxford University Press Inc., ISBN 978-0-19-953494-4, New York, United States

Shah J: (2002) Endoscopy through the ages, *BJU* 2002: 89:645-652

Sylvester RJ, Oosterlinck W & van der Meijden AP. (2004)   A single immediate postoperative instillation of chemotherapy decreases the risk of recurrence in patients with stage Ta T1 bladder cancer: a meta-analysis of published results of randomized clinical trials *J Urol* 171(6 pt 1) June 2004: pp 2186-2190.

Turk, C.; Knoll, T.; Petrik, A.; Sarica, K.; Seitz, C.; Straub, M.; Traxer, O. (2010). *Guidelines on Urolithiasis*, EAU (European Association of Urology 2010)

Part 3

Pediatric Endoscopy

6

Diagnostic and Therapeutic Sinonasal Endoscopy in Pediatric Patients

Marco Berlucchi[1], Barbara Pedruzzi[1],
Michele Sessa[2] and Piero Nicolai[2]
[1]Department of Pediatric Otorhinolaryngology,
Spedali Civili, Brescia
[2]Department of Otolaryngology,
University of Brescia, Brescia
Italy

1. Introduction

Fifty years ago, the extracorporeal cold light and its transmission by glass fibers, along with the Hopkins rod lens system, were introduced. The development and application of these new technologies to upper airways allowed studying, understanding, and improving knowledge of the anatomy, physiology, and diseases of the nasal cavity and sinuses. In particular, some fundamental concepts of modern rhinology are based on endoscopic nasal findings and Messerklinger's investigations of the pathophysiology of sinus mucosa. These studies radically changed traditional understanding of sinus inflammation and revolutionized its treatment using endoscopic conservative surgical management (Messerklinger, 1966, 1967, 1978). In the 1980s, Kennedy (Kennedy, 1985) first utilized this surgical technique in the United States and termed it functional endoscopic sinus surgery (FESS). At the beginning, the technique was performed only for treatment of rhinosinusitis in adult patients. In following years, the surgical indications were extended to selected malignant neoplasms (Kennedy & Senior, 1997; Lund, 1997; Nicolai et al., 2009, 2011). Due to the good results observed by FESS, in 1990s the development of smaller endoscopes and instrumentation adapted for pediatric patients was encouraged. For the treatment of recurrent or chronic rhinosinusitis in children, favorable results were obtained with endoscopic surgery (Lusk & Muntz, 1990; Wolf et al., 1995). During subsequent years, other diseases of sinuses were treated successfully with a nasal endoscopic surgical approach (Triglia & Nicollas, 1997: Berlucchi et al., 2003, 2010; Woodworth et al., 2004; Nicollas et al., 2006; Durmaz et al., 2008; Al-Mazrou et al., 2009; Presutti et al., 2009; Nicolai et al., 2010). In this chapter, a description of endonasal diagnostic techniques and a brief report of sinonasal disorders that may be effectively treated by FESS in pediatric patients are presented. Finally, fundamental surgical steps and their relation between pediatric endoscopic sinus surgery (PESS) and facial growth is briefly discussed.

2. Diagnostic nasal endoscopic procedures

The availability of adequate equipment such as flexible and rigid nasal endoscopes of various degrees and sizes (Fig. 1,2,3) is fundamental to achieve accurate endonasal diagnoses.

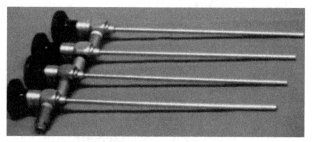

Fig. 1. Nasal rigid endoscopes.

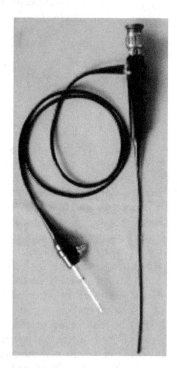

Fig. 2. Flexible endoscope.

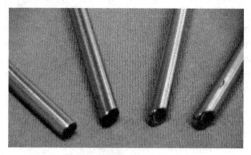

Fig. 3. Tips of the rigid nasal endoscopes of various degrees.

The choice of nasal endoscope is related to the age and compliance of the pediatric patient. In compliant children and in those older than 8 years, 4-mm and/or 2.7-mm rigid nasal endoscopes are usually well tolerated and provide good endoscopic nasal views. Because of possible traumatic complications, in non-compliant children and in those younger than 8 years, 3.5-mm and/or 2.5 mm flexible endoscopes must be utilized even if they provide an endonasal vision that is qualitatively inferior compared to rigid endoscopes. Before performing nasal endoscopy, cottons soaked with decongestant and local anesthetic are placed in the nasal cavities for about 10 minutes. This allows simultaneously augmenting the space of nasal fossae and obtaining a topical anesthetic effect. This may be easily performed in adolescents, whereas in toddlers and non-compliant children a local anesthetic is preferable sprayed in the nasal cavities. In infants and neonates, topical drugs are not generally utilized. During rhinoscopy, the child is placed in either a sitting position or kept in the arms of a nurse in relation to age and compliance. Nasal endoscopy must be performed correctly, meticulously, and accurately to avoid traumatic lesions of endonasal structures. Before starting endoscopic evaluation, whenever possible it is important to explain the diagnostic procedure to the child in the attempt to obtain full collaboration. After removal of cottonoids and treatment of the endoscopic lens with a thin film of anti-fog solution, the endoscope is inserted slowly and delicately in the nasal fossa. First, the floor of the nose and nasal septum, inferior nasal turbinate and its meatus are examined (Fig. 4).

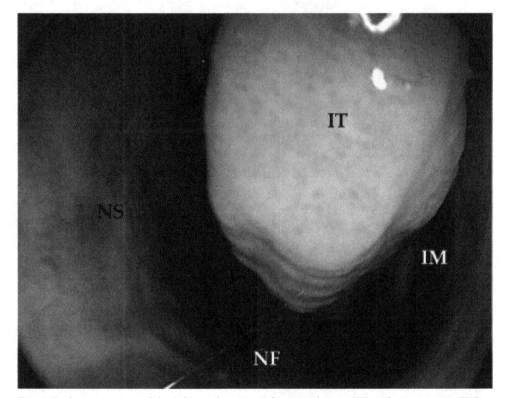

Fig. 4. Endoscopic view of the left nasal cavity: inferior turbinate (IT), inferior meatus (IM), nasal septum (NS), and nasal floor (NF).

Advancing posteriorly, the entire nasopharynx, Eustachian tube orifices, and torus tubarius can be assessed (Fig. 5).

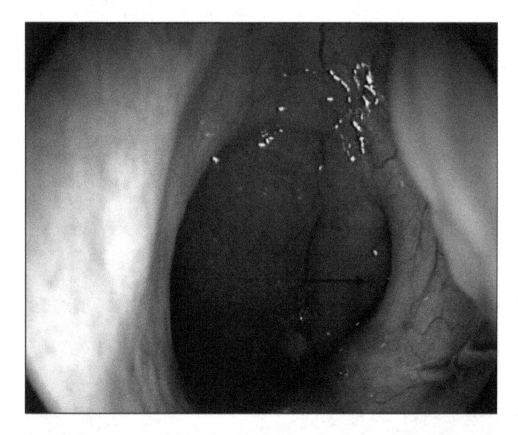

Fig. 5. Nasopharynx and left Eustachian tube orifice (arrow) at endoscopic evaluation.

Afterwards, coming back and turning the endoscope superiorly, the middle nasal turbinate and its meatus are explored (Fig. 6).

When the endoscope moves toward the uncinate process area, fontanellae, accessory maxillary sinus ostia, and sphenoethmoid recess can be assessed. By rotating the endoscope superiorly when it is located anteriorly to the head of middle turbinate, it is possible to observe the anterior olfactory region. In addition to evaluation of nasal anatomy, rhinoscopy allows assessment of mucosa status, the presence and type of endonasal secretions (i.e., serous, mucous, or purulent discharge) and their suspicious origin, associated disorders, and their relationships with surrounding structures. Furthermore, rhinoscopy allows monitoring sinonasal diseases such as rhinosinusitis and adenoid hypertrophy, as well as postsurgical follow-up of nasal sinuses. It can also evaluate response to medical treatment, ease cavity debridement in the post-operative period to favor healing of the sinuses, and identify persistent or early recurrences of sinonasal lesions.

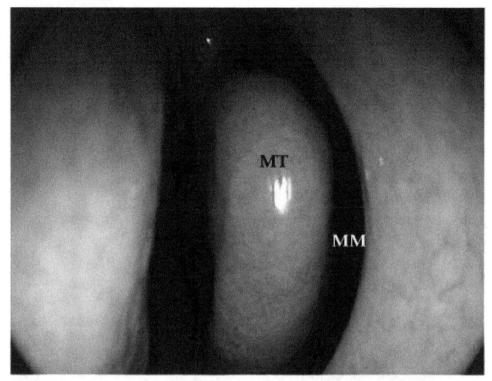

Fig. 6. Endoscopic examination of the head of the middle turbinate (MT) and middle meatus (MM).

3. Sinonasal disorders treated by endoscopic sinonasal surgery

Numerous sinonasal diseases can be successfully treated by endoscopic sinus surgery. Extensive surgical experience is mandatory to treat some sinonasal lesions and to obtain good results. Several sinonasal pathologies will be briefly discussed.

3.1 Inferior turbinate hypertrophy

Inferior turbinate hypertrophy can be either congenital or acquired. The former is rare, whereas the latter is usually due to septal deviation, allergic rhinitis, or gastroesophageal reflux disease (Kwok et al., 2007; Cingi et al., 2010). The primary presenting symptom is nasal obstruction occasionally associated with seromucosal rhinorrhea, itching, and sneezing. Moreover, chronic nasal obstruction may modify the normal function of the Eustachian tube causing effusion in the middle ear (Pelikan, 2009). Diagnosis is made by nasal endoscopy. Rhinomanometry in basal conditions and after decongestion can be added in selected cases.

3.2 Adenoid hypertrophy

Adenoid hypertrophy is probably the most frequent pathology in the pediatric population. This disorder manifests usually between 3 and 6 years of age in both sexes. Children complain of bilateral nasal obstruction associated with snoring, rhinorrhea, mouth breathing, hyponasal speech, and cough (Berlucchi et al., 2007). In some cases, obstructive sleep apnea syndrome can also be observed. The pathology may lead to cardiorespiratory syndromes such as cor pulmonale in extreme cases. Furthermore, adenoid hypertrophy may favor other illnesses such as recurrent and effusive otitis media and recurrent/chronic rhinosinusitis. Nasal endoscopy is the gold standard diagnostic technique to evaluate adenoid size, inflammatory and infectious status, and its anatomical relationship with the nasopharyngeal orifice of Eustachian tubes. Moreover, it allows checking changes in adenoid size after medical therapy (Cassano et al., 2003; Berlucchi et al., 2007). At endoscopic assessment, adenoids appear as a single pyramid-shaped aggregation of lymphoid tissue with the apex pointed toward the nasal septum and the base at the level of the superior and posterior wall of the nasopharynx. The adenoid pad appears as a lobulated and pinkish mass, partially or totally occupying the nasopharynx (Fig. 7).

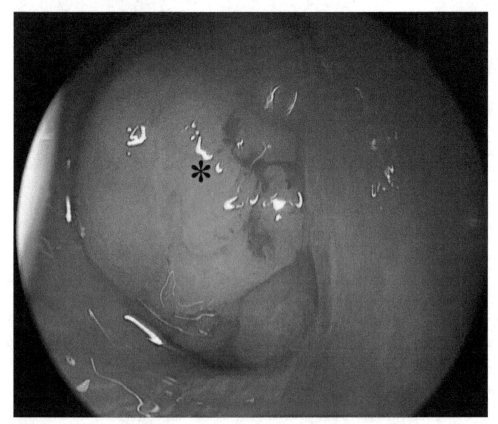

Fig. 7. Adenoid hypertrophy (asterisk) totally obstructing the right nasal fossa.

3.3 Sinonasal polyposis
Sinonasal polyposis is an uncommon pathology in pediatric subjects (Triglia & Nicollas, 1997). In the 1990s, the disorder was classified in 5 subtypes: antrochoanal polyps (this

lesion will be described separately due to its peculiar characteristics), choanal polyps, polyps associated with chronic rinosinusitis (non-eosinophil dominated), polyps associated with chronic rinosinusitis (eosinophil dominated), and polyps associated with specific illnesses such as cystic fibrosis, Kartagener's Syndrome, and asthma (Stammberger, 1999). Even though the etiology of sinonasal polyposis is unknown, some predisposing factors have been identified. The lesions affect both sexes and can be either monolateral or bilateral. Clinically, children complain of nasal obstruction, rhinorrhea, reduction of the sense of smell or anosmia, headache, and facial pain (Triglia & Nicollas, 1997). At nasal endoscopy, polyps show a characteristic edematous and translucid appearance (Fig. 8).

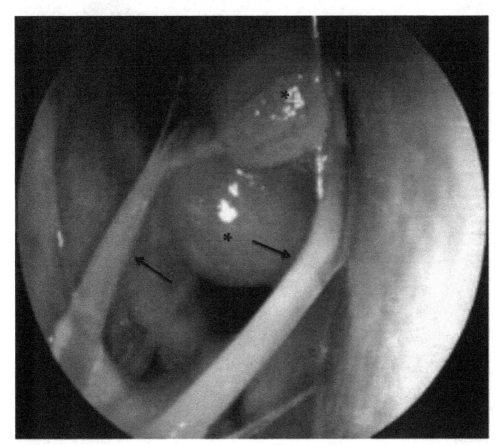

Fig. 8. Nasal polyps (asterisks) associated with mucous secretion (arrows) in a patient with cystic fibrosis.

They can fill partially or totally the nasal cavity and may be associated with a broad or narrow pedicle. Imaging is the diagnostic technique of choice, and CT of the sinuses is the gold standard procedure as it shows exact extension of disease and presence of anatomic anomalies, which may favor sinonasal polyps and/or influence surgical strategy (Triglia & Nicollas, 1997).

3.4 Antrochoanal polyp

First described by Paefyn in 1753 (Paefyn, 1753), antrochoanal polyp (ACP) or Killian's polyp is a benign, solitary, nasal polypoid lesion. It represents 4-6% of all nasal polyps in the general population (Yaman et al., 2010). It is also is prevalent in the pediatric age, and ACP is found in about one-third of pediatric cases with polyps (Schramm & Effron, 1980; Basak et al., 1998; Ozdek et al., 2002; Yaman et al., 2010). The mass originates inside the maxillary sinus and as it grows it extends from the accessory or natural ostium of maxillary sinus to the middle meatus (Fig. 9), finally protruding toward the choana in the nasopharynx.

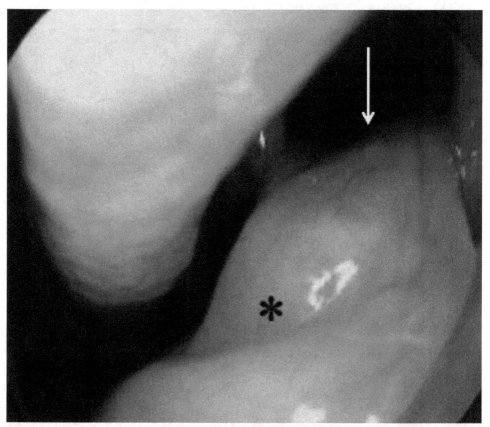

Fig. 9. Left antrochoanal polyp (asterisk) that come out from natural ostium (white arrow) of maxillary sinus.

From an etiological point of view, ACP develops from intramural Tornwaldt's cyst in the wall of the maxillary sinus. This particular origin reflects the presence of cysts in the antral portion of the polyp (Berg et al., 1988; Skladzień, 2001). Chronic sinus inflammation and allergy are other factors favoring formation of ACP (Skladzień et al., 2001). The disorder, whose etiology is still unknown, is usually unilateral and more frequent in males (M:F=2.1:1). ACP is composed of cystic and solid portions. The former occupies the maxillary sinus, while the latter, which generally emerges through an enlarged maxillary accessory ostium, is found in the nasal fossa. The most common symptoms are unilateral nasal obstruction, rhinorrhea, bleeding, headache, snoring, and foreign body sensation (Orvidas et al., 2001; Aydil et al., 2008). Moreover, in 20-25% of cases nasal obstruction may be bilateral, in relation to complete blockage of the nasopharynx. Moreover, some reports have described dysphagia and dyspnea correlated with mouth extension. Nasal endoscopy and CT are the gold standard diagnostic procedures. At endoscopic examination, the lesion appears as a white and bright mass located in the middle meatus. This mass juts out the maxillary sinus and occupies the nasal fossa (Frosini et al., 2009). At imaging, ACP fills the maxillary sinus growing through the accessory or natural ostium into the middle meatus to the choana (Pruna et al., 2000). By MR, the lesion reveals hypointense T1 and enhanced T2 signals, and the cystic part is enhanced in the peripheral area after intravenous gadolinium administration (De Vuysere et al., 2001).

3.5 CSF leak

Cerebrospinal fluid (CSF) leak occurs when there is abnormal communication between the space containing CSF around the brain (subarachnoid space) and the sinonasal tract and/or the ear (middle ear/mastoid system) (Pianta et al., 2005). It implies a breach of the underlying dura mater and adherent pia-arachnoid mater resulting in a pathological communication between the intracranial cavity and either the nasal or middle ear cavity (Lloyd et al., 2008; Presutti et al., 2009). According to Ommaya's classification (Ommaya, 1976), CSF leaks can be divided into non-traumatic (with high or normal CSF pressure) and traumatic (accidental or iatrogenic lesion). About 80% and 16% of CSF leaks are due to head trauma and sinuses or skull base surgery, respectively (Beckhardt et al., 1991). Spontaneous fistulae, which are more frequent in obese females in the fourth decade of life (Pianta et al., 2005), represent 3–4% of cases (Beckhardt et al., 1991; Yerkes et al., 1992; Nachtigal et al., 1999; Schlosser & Bolger, 2002). Moreover, skull base tumors or other congenital lesions (such as untreated aqueductal stenosis) may cause CSF leaks directly through erosion of the skull base or indirectly through the development of hydrocephalus. Other congenital causes of CSF leak are the developmental of skull base defects with associated meningoceles, meningoencephaloceles, large arachnoid granulations or cysts, or congenital inner ear anomalies (Lloyd et al., 2008). If the pathogenesis of traumatic fistula is intuitive, spontaneous leaks may have a multifactorial origin. Among these, intracranial pressure, brain pulsation, cranial base pneumatization, and arachnoid pits are thought to play a major role (Pianta et al., 2005). Spontaneous CSF fistula occurs commonly at the ethmoid roof, cribriform plate, perisella of sphenoid sinus, or inferolateral or pterygoid recess (Lloyd et al., 2008). Patients with CFS leak suffer from unilateral or bilateral watery persistent or intermittent rhinorrhea with positive history for a previous head trauma or surgery of the sinonasal tract, middle ear/mastoid, or skull base. Increase of postnasal drip in the supine position may be reported. Moreover, patients can complain of a salty or sweet taste in the mouth. Recurrent meningitis should alert the physician to a diagnosis of CSF leak (Pianta et al., 2005). Intermittent clear nasal discharge may be exacerbated by the Valsalva maneuver and/or compression of both internal jugular veins (Pianta et al., 2005). When the lesion is located in the temporal bone, CSF reaches the nasopharynxc via the Eustachian tube and becomes evident in most cases as bilateral clear rhinorrhea (Pianta et al., 2005). Patients with intermittent CSF leak complain frequently of headache, which appears whenever rhinorrhea stops and the CSF pressure increases (Beckhardt et al., 1991). Finally, signs and symptoms such as headache, vomit, or edema of the papilla are suggestive for intracranial hypertension (Pianta et al., 2005). "Reservoir sign" is a feature suggestive for the presence of a CSF fistula at the sphenoid, and is due to accumulation of CSF in the sphenoid sinus when the patient is recumbent. It remains in the sinus until the patient resumes an erect position and the head is leaned forward. At that moment, fluid exits from sphenoid ostium and sudden profuse rhinorrhea becomes evident (Nuss & Costantino, 1995). Diagnosis of CSF leak includes laboratory testing, imaging, and fluorescein test. The former includes dosage of several proteins (i.e., beta-2 transferrin or beta-trace protein) on the watery fluid collected from the nose. These are polypeptides produced in the brain, leptomeninges, or choroid plexus that may be identified in nasal mucus when CFS leak is present (Bachmann et al., 2000; Lloyd et al., 2008). Radiological procedures such as CT and MR are used to localize and characterize the involved site, to evaluate for an underlying cause, and to exclude an associated meningocele or meningoencephalocele (Lloyd et al., 2008). Finally, fluorescein test is performed by intra- or peri-operative intrathecal injection of dye solution diluted with 10 ml of CFS (Pianta et al., 2005). This can allow localization of the site of leak and ensure successful closure during surgical intervention.

3.6 Rhinosinusitis

As rhinitis and sinusitis are usually simultaneous, the use of the term rhinosinusitis is medically correct. This disorder is a common upper airway infection in the pediatric age. It is an inflammation of nasal cavity and sinuses and is characterized by two o more symptoms one of which should be either nasal obstruction or nasal discharge associated or no with facial pain/pressure and reduction or loss of smell. Based on duration of symptomatology, rhinosinusitis can be divided into: 1) acute rhinosinusitis, when total resolution of aforementioned symptoms may take up to 12 weeks; 2) chronic rhinosinusitis, when clinical picture persists for more than 12 weeks; and 3) recurrent acute rhinosinusitis, when multiple acute rhinosinusitis occurs with total resolution of each acute episode (Fokkens et al., 2007). Several predisposing factors such as allergy, adenoid mass, gastroesophageal reflux disease, sinonasal anomalies (i.e., septal deviation, concha bullosa, Haller cell, choanal atresia, and paradoxical middle turbinate), immunological disorders, primary ciliary dyskinesia, cystic fibrosis, exposure to tobacco, and daycare attendance have been noted to favor rhinosinusitis (Lusk, 1992, 1997; Clement 2008). The classical triad, which is generally responsible for upper respiratory infections (i.e., *Streptococcus pneumoniae, Haemophilus influenzae, and Moraxella catarrhalis*), has been shown to be involved in most acute rhinosinusitis as well. *Staphylococcus aureus* and *anaerobes* can be occasionally found (Lieser & Derkay 2005). Clinically, rhinosinusitis is characterized by rhinorrhea, nasal obstruction, cough, headache, and facial pain. Purulent rhinorrhea, periorbital edema, and high fever may be observed in severe form. Signs and symptoms of chronic rhinosinusitis are those of the non-severe acute form, but they persist for more than 12 weeks. At rhinoscopy, diffuse mucosal inflammation associated with turbinate congestion is the typical endonasal endoscopic appearance of acute rhinosinusitis (Fig. 10).

Mucopurulent secretions can be also present and, in relation to their site, it is possible to suspect which sinuses may be affected. Purulent secretions located at middle meatus or sphenoethmoid recess are a sign of involvement of maxillary, ethmoid, and/or frontal sinus and sphenoid sinus, respectively. Under endoscopic control, cultures can be taken directly

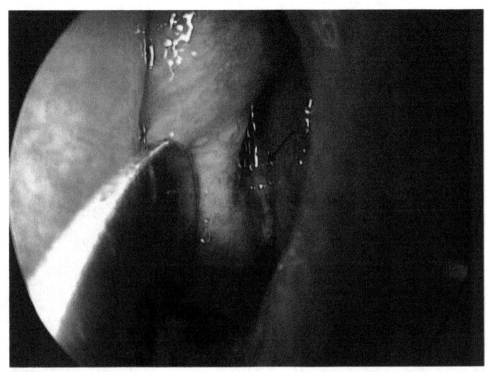

Fig. 10. Diffuse nasal mucosal inflammation and congestion of middle turbinate. After medial dislocation of middle turbinate, purulent secretion is found in the middle meatus (arrow).

from the involved meatus. Polypoid changes around the middle turbinate insertion is indicative of inflammation of the frontal sinus, whereas the presence of polyps suggests chronic rhinosinusitis (Joe et al., 2001). Moreover, nasal endoscopy allows monitoring inflammation and objectively evaluating the response to treatment. For this reason, serial endoscopic nasal examinations are mandatory to individualize therapy and, eventually, to modify antibiotic administration when no improvement is observed. Diagnosis is based on careful assessment of the patient's history and clinical picture. In dubious cases, endoscopy of nasal cavity can confirm clinical suspicion. Microbiological cultures are not routinely necessary, but when sinus infection does not improve using antibiotic therapy within 48-72 hours, occurs in an immunocompromised patient, the child is toxic or extremely ill, suppurative complications are evident, or when infectious sinonasal illness recurs 1-2 weeks after the end of medical therapy, microbiological evaluation is mandatory (Lusk & Stankiewicz, 1997; Clement, 2008). Imaging is not indicated to confirm a diagnosis of rhinosinusitis. CT is performed after failure of medical therapy and, therefore, in the planning of surgery or when surgical treatment may be considered as in the aforementioned pathological situations (Lusk & Stankiewicz, 1997). Furthermore, examinations for allergy, cystic fibrosis, immunological disease, gastroesophageal reflux, and primary ciliary dyskinesia can be performed as necessary.

3.7 Choanal atresia

Choanal atresia (CA) is a rare, congenital disease characterized by complete obstruction of the posterior nasal passages. Its incidence is 1:5000-8000 live births (Teissier et al., 2008).

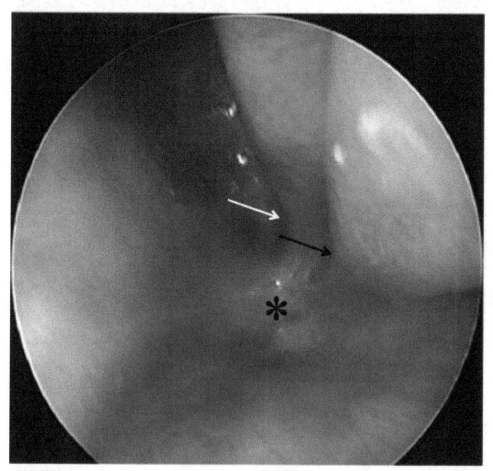

Fig. 11. Endoscopic view of the left choanal atresia (asterisk). The inferior turbinate (black arrow) and middle turbinate (white arrow) are also evident.

There is a female predominance with a F/M ratio of 5/1 among Caucasians. The lesion may be unilateral (60%) or bilateral (40%) and can subdivided into bony (90%) or membranous (10%) types (Vatansever et al., 2005). The genetic aspect of CA remains unclear and is likely multifactorial. In 50% of patients, CA is associated with other anomalies as in the CHARGE syndrome (coloboma, heart abnormalities, CA, retarded growth and development of central nervous system, genitourinary anomalies, ear defects) (Jyonouchi et al., 2009). Several theories such as persistence of the buccopharyngeal membranes, failure of the oronasal membrane to rupture either the nasobuccal membrane of Hochstetter or buccopharyngeal membrane of the foregut, incomplete resorption of nasopharyngeal mesoderm, or locally misdirected mesodermal flow have been proposed to explain the occurrence of CA, but none have been universally accepted. This process occurs between the 4th and 11th fetal week (Dunham & Miller, 1992; Keller & Kacker, 2000; Samadi et al., 2003). Since neonates are obligate nasal breathing, at birth bilateral choanal atresia can manifest with dyspnea, cyanosis, severe hypoxia, and suckling difficulties, whereas the unilateral form presents monolateral rhinorrhea. Its diagnosis can be late and, often, occasional. Endoscopic examination with flexible nasal endoscope is mandatory when CA is suspected. Endonasal evaluation shows complete closure of involved choana that may be associated with inflammation of nasal mucosa and mucous stagnation (Fig. 11).

Imaging is the next, fundamental diagnostic procedure. CT performed in axial and coronal projections provides a thorough assessment of CA, reveals the bony or membranous nature of the disease, and shows the narrowing of posterior nasal cavity and the thickening of the vomer (Schweinfurth, 2002).

3.8 Mucocele

Mucocele is a benign, cyst-like, locally expansile paranasal sinus mass. The pathology consists of accumulation of secretion products, aseptic slimy mucus, desquamation, and inflammation lined by the respiratory mucosa (Marks et al., 1997; Busaba & Salman, 1999), developing within a paranasal sinus associated with expansion of its bony walls as a consequence of ostium blockage. A mucocele grows slowly and expands by eroding the surrounding bony walls. The obstruction can result from congenital anomalies, chronic rhinosinusitis, previous radiotherapy and/or surgical treatment, trauma, and sinonasal neoplasms (Johnson & Ferguson, 1998; Maroldi et al., 2005). Moreover, congenital illnesses such as cystic fibrosis and primary ciliary dyskinesia are considered predisposing factors for occurrence of mucoceles (Guttenplan & Wetmore, 1989; Thomé et al., 2000; Nicollas et al., 2006; Olze et al., 2006; Berlucchi et al., 2010). Mucoceles occur more frequently in the fourth and fifth decade of life, with a similar distribution in both sexes. Paranasal sinuses mucoceles are extremely rare in a pediatric age and most cases described have been associated with cystic fibrosis (Olze et al., 2006). The frontal sinus is involved in 60% of cases, followed by the ethmoid labyrinth and maxillary sinus with 30% and less than 10% of cases, respectively. Few cases are localized in the sphenoid sinus (Som & Brandwein, 1996; Arruè et al., 1998; Lloyd et al., 2000; Caylakli et al., 2006). The higher incidence of mucoceles in the frontal sinus seems to be related to anatomical variations of the frontal recess (Arruè et al., 1998; Martin et al., 2000). Mucoceles are usually monolateral, whereas bilateral mucoceles are infrequently observed (Varghese et al., 2004). The clinical picture, which varies in relation to the sinus involved, includes nasal obstruction, rhinorrhea, headache, cheek pressure or pain associated with or without check swelling, maxillary nerve hyperesthesia, infra-orbital anesthesia, dental pain, loosening of teeth, periorbital pain, proptosis, blurred vision, alteration of visual acuity, diplopia, and sudden loss of vision (Avery et al., 1983; Hayasaka et al., 1991; Moriyama et al., 1992; Curtin & Rabinov, 1998; Busaba & Salman 1999; Maroldi et al., 2005; Tseng et al., 2005). Whenever erosion of the anterior or posterior wall of the frontal sinus is present, a Pott's puffy tumor or neurological symptoms may be evident (Maroldi et al., 2005). At nasal endoscopy, the appearance varies according to the site of the mucocele and the phase of growth. During the intrasinusal phase, no alterations are generally visible. The subsequent expansion of the mucocele may alter the paranasal sinus bony walls. In a maxillary localization, medialization of the middle turbinate, anterior dislocation of the uncinate process (Fig. 12),

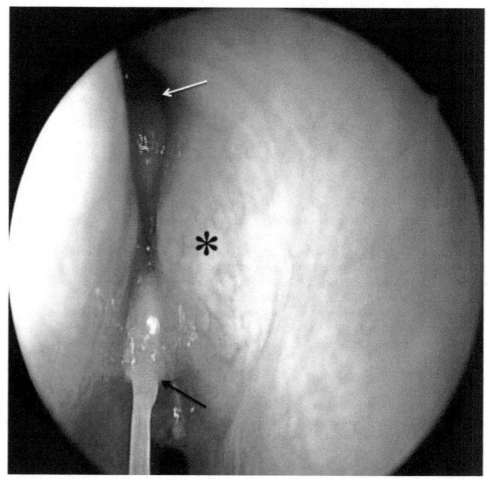

Fig. 12. Anterior displacement of the left uncinate process (asterisk) due to mucocele of the maxillary sinus at endoscopic examination. Mucous secretion (black arrow) and middle turbinate (white arrow) are also observed.

and bulging of the agger nasi cells or the infundibular area can be observed, whereas submucosal remodeling or bulging of the sphenoethmoid recess or posterior ethmoid can be evident in sphenoidal mucoceles. In frontal mucoceles, endoscopic examination is usually negative (Maroldi et al., 2005) since the lesion has expanded inferiorly to involve the agger nasi. Diagnosis is based on signs and symptoms, nasal endoscopic evaluation, and imaging. By CT, the disease appears as a homogenous lesion that completely occupies the involved sinus with smooth clear-cut margins of bone erosion of its walls (Han et al., 1995; Busaba & Salman, 1999). Moreover, CT shows the site and extension of the disease, remolded cortex, bony erosion entity, anatomical variants, and hyperostotic changes, (Maroldi et al., 2005). MR is usually performed when mucocele formation is secondary to sinonasal soft tissue tumors in which the lining membrane of the mucocele will enhance after intravenous contrast (Jayaraj et al., 1999).

3.9 Meningoencephalocele

Cephalocele or encephalocele (EC) is an extracranial extension of any intracranial structure through a congenital or acquired defect of the skull base (Pianta et al., 2005). Such herniation may be represented by the leptomeninges associated with cerebrospinal fluid or it can also include the brain. The former is defined meningocele (MC), whereas the latter is termed meningoencephalocele (MEC) (Naidich et al., 1992). The incidence of EC ranges from 1 case/5,000 live births in Thailand to about 1 case/40,000 live births in western countries (Mahapatra & Suri, 2002). The disorder may be divided into occipital, parietal, basal, and syncipital types (Mc Carty et al., 1990). The latter group is subdivided into fronto-ethmoidal and interfrontal subtypes, and those associated with craniofacial clefts (C. Suwanwela & N. Suwanwela, 1972). The fronto-ethmoidal form, which accounts for about 10% of all meningoceles, includes: 1) naso-ethmoidal form that is the herniation of meninges with or without brain tissue through the anterior cranial base at the level of the foramen caecum between nasal bone and nasal cartilage; 2) naso-frontal form that occurs between nasal and frontal bones; and 3) naso-orbital form that develops between the maxilla and lacrimal bones. MEC is located at the occipital region in 75% of cases, followed in order of frequency by the frontoethmoidal and parietal area in about 15% and 10% of patients, respectively. (Hoving, 2000; Mahapatra & Aqrawal, 2006). The neural tissue in MEC was initially considered dysplastic and non-functioning, but since functioning brain has been found in some occipital and trans-sphenoidal MEC, this concept has been recently revisited (Pianta et al., 2005). MEC may cause nasal obstruction and CSF rhinorrhea. This latter symptom can be unilateral or bilateral, persistent or intermittent, and it increases or may be elicited by maneuvers elevating CSF pressure such as compression of the internal jugular veins or the Valsalva maneuver (Pianta et al., 2005). Moreover, MEC can promote alterations and distortions of surrounding facial structures such as displacement of the medial orbital wall, orbit, telecanthus, broad nasal bridge, nasal and/or glabellar swelling, and hypertelorism. Ocular and lacrimal signs and symptoms (i.e., decrease of visual acuity, strabismus, epiphora and/or dacryocystitis) can be observed (Lello et al., 1989; Morris et al., 1989). At nasal endoscopic evaluation, the lesion may appear as a smooth, isolated, pulsatile polypoid mass arising from the olfactory fossa or sphenoid sinus (Samii & Draf 1989; Pianta et al., 2005). The site of the lesion may increase upon jugular vein compression (Furstenberg sign). In addition to evaluation of the clinical picture and nasal endoscopy, diagnostic work-up of MEC must include imaging. CT can show bony defects of the craniofacial junction and the sclerotic margins of the bone defect (Pianta et al., 2005), whereas MR may reveal the relationship with brain.

3.10 Lacrimal duct stenosis

With an incidence ranging from 6 to 84%, congenital lacrimal duct obstruction is a common disorder at birth. Fortunately, most cases resolve spontaneously within the first months of life. The remaining patients will require conservative procedures (lacrimal probing and intubation) and, if symptomatology persists, non-conservative management (dacryocystorhinostomy) will be performed (Berlucchi et al., 2003). The pathology is due to lack of canalization of the lacrimal system that generally intervenes at the distal end (Hasner's valve). Epiphora and recurrent dacryocystitis represent the typical clinical picture observed. Rarely, some patients present bulging of the medial canthus that corresponds to dacryocystocele. This cystic lesion of the lacrimal sac is due to both proximal (Rosenmuller's valve) and distal (Hasner's valve) obstruction. When the lesion expands in the nasal fossa at the level of inferior meatus (Fig. 13), the patient may also complain of different degrees of nasal obstruction in relation to its size (Wong & VanderVeen, 2008); respiratory distress can also be observed in bilateral localization.

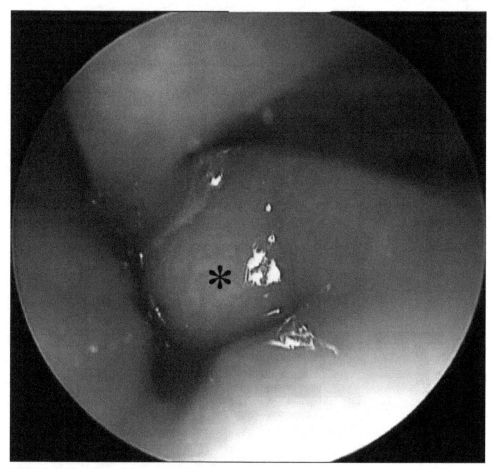

Fig. 13. Endoscopic view of a nasolacrimal duct cyst (asterisk).

At nasal endoscopy, the nasal cavity can be completely normal or, in some cases, a nasolacrimal duct cyst can be identified in the inferior meatus. Ophthalmologic and otorhinolaryngologic evaluation, dacryocystography, and CT of sinuses are the diagnostic procedures indicated or required (Berlucchi et al., 2003).

3.11 Lobular capillary hemangioma

Also known as pyogenic granuloma, telengiectasic granuloma, granuloma pedunculatum, and infected granuloma, lobular capillary hemangioma (LCH) is a benign, rapidly growing, painless, easily-bleeding, solitary lesion, which occurs in the skin and mucous membranes (Maroldi et al., 2005). Although several factors (i.e., nasal trauma, hormonal influences, viral oncogenes, underlying microscopic arteriovenous malformations, and the production of angiogenic growth factors) have been advocated to favor this disorder, its etiopathogenesis remains unknown (Puxeddu et al., 2006). In the head and neck area, the lesion commonly occurs in the oral cavity (gingiva, lips, tongue, and buccal mucosa), whereas involvement of the nasal cavity is rare (Simo et al., 1998; Ozcan et al., 2004). Sinonasal localization ranges from 7% to 29%, and the lesion more frequently involves the anterior portion of the nasal septum and the tip of the turbinates (Maroldi et al., 2005). The disease most often occurs in the third decade of life, with a female predominance (El-Sayed & al-Serhani, 1997; Maroldi et al., 2005), whereas its occurrence in pediatric populations has been only rarely reported (Berlucchi et al., 2010). The most common symptoms of LCH of the nasal cavity are recurrent unilateral epistaxis, nasal obstruction, and nasal discharge; facial pain, hyposmia and alteration of smell, and headache are rarely present (Ozcan et al., 2004; Puxeddu et al. 2006). At nasal endoscopy, the lesion usually appears as a single reddish hypervascularized polypoid mass that bleeds easily (Fig. 14).

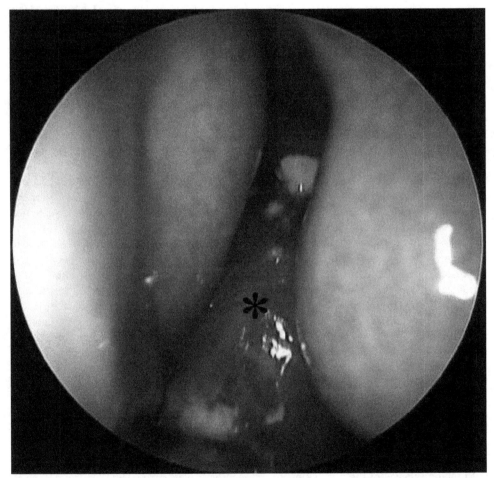

Fig. 14. Lobular capillary hemangioma (asterisk) completely occluding left nasal cavity.

When a nasal LCH is small, diagnosis is not difficult, while problems occur when the mass is relatively large and its macroscopic appearance is unclear. In these situations, imaging is mandatory (Berlucchi et al., 2010) as it reveals important features of the lesion such as size, probable site of origin, and vascularization pattern. CT shows a soft-tissue density nasal lesion with lobulated contours. MR reveals masses with an intermediate to hyperintense signal on T2-weighted images and a hypointense signal on T1-weighted images. Enhancement after contrast administration can be helpful (Berlucchi et al., 2010).

3.12 Nasal glioma

Nasal glioma (NG), also known as nasal glial heterotopias, brain-like heterotopia, glial hamartoma, heterotopic neuroglial tissue, nasal cerebral heterotopias, cephalic brain-like heterotopias, and nasal heterotopic brain tissue (Rahbar et al., 2003; Pakkasjärvi et al., 2008), is a rare benign developmental abnormality of neurogenic origin. The peak of occurrence is between 5 and 10 years of age, with a male-to-female ratio of 3:2 (Puppala et al., 1990; Vuckovic et al., 2006). The disorder represents 0.25% of all nasal tumors and accounts for approximately 5% of all congenital nasal swellings (Dabholkar et al., 2004, Vuckovic et al., 2006). The most widely accepted etiopathogenetic theory is that NG represents an encephalocele that becomes sequestered from the brain early in gestation. This is probably due to an abnormal closure of the nasal and frontal bone (fonticulus frontalis) that can lead to an ectopic remnant of glial tissue that remains extracranially (Ma & Keung, 2006). Since it is not a true neoplasm, the term NG is actually not correct. The lesion consists of ectopic/heterotopic neural tissue with neuroglial elements and glial cells in a matrix of connective tissue with or without a fibrous connection to the subarachnoid space or dura. It can grow within the nasal region and is covered by skin or respiratory mucosa (Lowe et al., 2000, Vuckovic 2006). Moreover, 90% of NG do not contain neurons and its benign nature is demonstrated by a low proliferative activity (Dimov et al., 2001). NG can be extranasal (60% of cases), lying external to the nasal bones and cavities; intranasal (30%), lying within the nasal cavity (Fig. 15), mouth, or pterygopalatine fossa; or mixed (10%), communicating through a defect of nasal bones. Extranasal gliomas that are usually paramedian are generally located at the glabella, but can be also present laterally or at the nasal tip (Uzunlar et al., 2001; Vuckovic et al., 2006). Intranasal lesions are usually located within the nasal passage medially to the middle turbinate bone. The intranasal type is more often associated with dural attachment (35%) than the extranasal type (9%) (Kennard & Rasmussen, 1990). Finally, combined intra/extranasal gliomas have a typical dumbbell shape with a connecting band (Vuckovic et al., 2006). Patients with NG may complain of nasal obstruction, epistaxis, and cerebrospinal fluid rhinorrhea. Moreover, the lesion can be associated with deformities of the adjacent bones and nasal cartilage such as widened nose and obstruction of the nasolacrimal duct. Hypertelorism, broadening of the nasal bridge, airway obstruction, and epiphora are secondary to growth of the mass (Bradley & Singh, 1982; Fitzpatrick & Miller, 1996). At endoscopic view, NGs appear as nonpulsatile, uncompressible, gray or reddish-blue to purple, soft or firm at touch, and polypoid-like lesion. The mass, which is present on the nasal dorsum and/or arises from the lateral nasal wall, may be associated with telangiectasias of the overlying skin (Hengerer & Newburg, 1990). Neuroimaging is mandatory to identify nasal lesions, to exclude its possible intracranial connection, and to plan the optimal surgical approach (Harley 1991; Hoeger et al., 2001). Because of its potential intracranial connection, excisional biopsy or fine needle aspiration cytology should not be performed due to the risk of meningitis or cerebrospinal fluid (CSF) leak (Claros 1998).

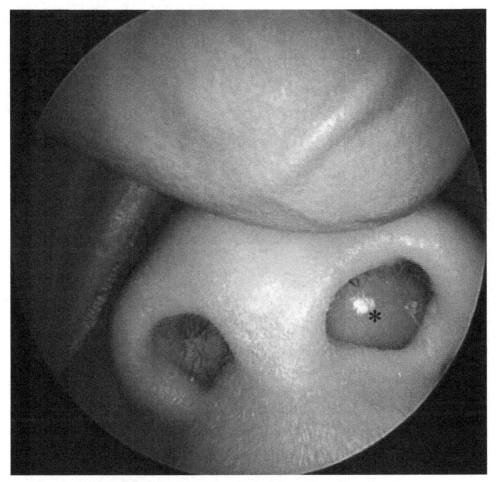

Fig. 15. Intranasal glioma (asterisk) occupying the left nasal pyriform aperture.

3.13 Juvenile angiofibroma

Juvenile angiofibroma (JA) is a highly vascular benign and locally invasive lesion that accounts around 0.05% of all head and neck neoplasms. The disorder typically occurs in adolescent males. Recently, some studies have reported that the lesion has an immunohistological and electron microscopic profile more consistent with a vascular malformation rather with a tumor (Beham et al., 1997, 2000). The site of origin of JA appears to be the sphenopalatine foramen or the bone of the vidian canal. From there, the lesion can expand to the nasopharynx, nasal fossa, paranasal sinuses, and pterygopalatine and infratemporal fossa. In some cases, involvement of the orbit and middle and anterior cranial fossa by bone erosion may be observed (Nicolai et al., 2003). Most patients present nasal obstruction associated with discharge and recurrent, spontaneous epistaxis. Due to enlargement of the tumor, facial swelling, proptosis, headache, cranial nerve palsies, and conductive hearing loss secondary to otitis media with effusion may also be observed. At nasal endoscopic evaluation, JA appears as sessile, lobulated, rubbery and red-pink to gray mass covered by several vascular structures (Fig. 16).

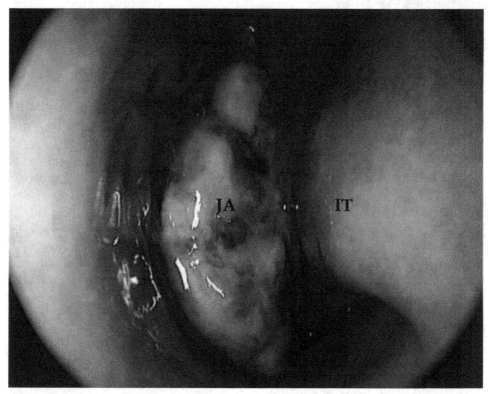

Fig. 16. Juvenile angiofibroma (JA) covered by several fibrin due a recent bleeding in the left nasal fossa. Inferior turbinate (IT).

It occupies usually the nasopharynx and nasal cavity, and it bleeds easily when touched. It may sometimes have a polypoid or pedunculated aspect. Because multiplanar evaluation of the disease and detailed information on the relationship between the lesion and important adjacent structures are needed, MR is considered the gold standard diagnostic procedure. Moreover, before surgical treatment, preoperative diagnostic assessment of the vascular pattern of the lesion by angiography is required, which should be associated with angiographic embolisation to decrease intraoperative bleeding and, consequently, the risk of perioperative transfusion (Nicolai et al., 2003). A biopsy of the lesion is not indicated due to profuse bleeding (Antonelli et al., 1987).

4. Surgical technique and its influence on facial growth

Before describing the main surgical procedures, it is fundamental to highlight some general aspects of PESS. 1) The patient must undergo preoperative CT of sinuses to evaluate anatomy, likely type of disease, and extension to plan surgical management. 2) Preoperative antibiotic and steroid therapy is also added to reduce inflammation and infection in the sinuses. 3) PESS is always performed under general anesthesia. 4) Endoscopes of different degrees (0°, 30°, 45°, and 70°) and size (4 and 2.7 mm), adult and pediatric instrumentation sets for PESS, and microdebrider must all be available in the operating room. 5) Application of cotton decongestant pledgets in nasal fossae for 10 minutes before surgical management is helpful to increase the nasal space. 6) Surgical management must be conservative and involves only the pathological sinuses. Herein, basal procedures about PESS are reported. Since extensive and advanced endoscopic sinus procedures are beyond the scope of the present chapter, these surgical treatments will not be presented.

4.1 Middle antrostomy
Submucosal injection of 1% mepivacaine chlorohydrate and 1:200,000 epinephrine is given at the level of the root of the middle turbinate and uncinate process. The posterior edge of uncinate process and, when evident, the main ostium of maxillary sinus are probed with a small seeker. Next, partial uncinectomy with conservation of its upper third is performed usually with back-biting forceps. When necessary, the natural ostium of the maxillary sinus can be wided both posteriorly and inferiorly. The risk-areas are nasolacrimal duct, sphenopalatine foramen, and lamina papyracea sited anteriorly, posteriorly, and superiorly, respectively.

4.2 Anterior and posterior ethmoidectomy
After removal of the uncinate process, the anterior wall of the ethmoid bulla is evident and may be opened. This surgical step may be performed by a microdebrider or Weil forceps, and must be achieved medially and inferiorly avoiding damage to the orbit and roof of sinus. At this point, basal lamella is exposed. When needed, the basal lamella is perforated by Weil forceps or microdebrider at the infero-medial portion to prevent damage to the lamina papyracea and fovea ethmoidalis which are situated laterally and superiorly, respectively. Next, each bony lamella is opened and removed. During this surgical step, the optic nerve, located posteriorly and superiorly, can be identified.

4.3 Sphenoidotomy
This is performed through transnasal, transethmoidal, or trans-septal approach, and the opening of sphenoid sinus is achieved only if the pathology involves this sinus. In this surgical procedure, instruments are utilized at an infero-medial angle to avoid injury of the optic nerve and internal carotid artery, which lie at the lateral wall of the sinus.

4.4 Frontal sinusotomy
Frontal sinusotomy is only rarely performed in pediatric patients as sinusotomy of the frontal sinus is highly challenging due to its small recess and anatomical position. A standard anterior ethmoidectomy associated with opening of agger nasi is usually sufficient to identify the frontal recess. If necessary, it can be enlarged using angle circular-biting forceps. It is mandatory do not to strip mucosa to avoid a secondary frontal stenosis.

4.5 Potential effects of PESS on midfacial and sinus development
Even though the use of PESS is diffuse worldwide, its potential effects on sinus development and midfacial growth are still object of discussion. In 1995, Wolf et al.

reviewed 124 children undergoing PESS for chronic recurrent rhinosinusitis. The mean age of patients was 12 years, with 3 children under 5 years. Based on a questionnaire about patient satisfaction and symptomatic relief, it was found that endoscopic surgical sinus surgery had no clinically relevant effects on facial bone development. In our opinion, these results might be influenced by the fact that only 25% of patients were under the age of 5 years, an age during which there is rapid growth of the sinuses. In 1996, Kosko et al. described 5 children who underwent PESS for recurrent rhinosinusitis at a median age of 30 months. After a mean follow-up of 42 months, these patients still complained of signs and symptoms of recurrent rhinosinusitis. For this reason, CT was performed in all children. Imaging revealed maxillary sinus hypoplasia in all patients without clinically apparent facial asymmetry. The authors concluded that this radiological finding might be related to endoscopic sinus surgery. In 2000, Senior et al. assessed the quantitative long-term impact of PESS on sinus development. In this study, 8 children who underwent PESS for periorbital or orbital sinusitis were reviewed after a mean follow-up of 6.9 years. Control groups included 9 adults without signs of rhinosinusitis on imaging and 10 adult patients with a clinical history of childhood sinus symptoms and CT-positive for rhinosinusitis. No significant differences in sinus volumes were observed among groups. In 2002, Bothwell et al. analyzed the long-term outcome of facial growth after PESS in a retrospective age-matched study. The study and control groups included 46 children who underwent PESS for chronic rhinosinusitis and 21 children who did not undergo intervention, respectively. Quantitative anthropomorphic and qualitative analyses were performed in all cases. No statistical differences in facial growth were identified between the two patient groups.

In 2006, Van Peteghem & Clement evaluated the influence of PESS on facial growth in a prospective study. The patient cohort consisted of 23 children with cystic fibrosis of whom 13 underwent endonasal surgical treatment for massive nasal polyposis. After a follow-up of at least 10 years, cephalometric measurements were performed in the surgical patients and compared with those obtained in non-surgical group. No significant differences were found. Thus, even if the available evidence seems to indicate that PESS does not significantly affect growth and development of sinuses, analysis of potential surgical effects during rapid growth on facial skeleton has not been well assessed and warrants further investigation.

5. Conclusion

The introduction of rigid and flexible endoscopes has radically changed both diagnosis and therapeutic approaches to sinonasal diseases in pediatric patients. Endoscopy of the nasal cavities and nasopharynx permits observation of important anatomical areas that were previously not visible, evaluating macroscopic characteristics of the sinonasal lesions and their relationship with the endonasal structures. When associated with imaging of the sinuses, it may influence therapeutic planning. Consecutive endoscopic nasal procedures can also monitor sinonasal illnesses and their response to medical therapy. Subsequent development of PESS permitted the possibility to perform targeted and conservative treatments. In the post-operative period, rhinoscopy facilitates accurate debridement of nasal fossae and sinuses, promoting their healing. Finally, the performance of regular endoscopic nasal follow-up may identify early recurrences of sinonasal pathologies.

6. References

Al-Mazrou, K.A.; Al-Qahtani, A. & AL-Fayez, A.L. (2009). Effectiveness of transnasal endoscopic powered adenoidectomy in patients with choanal adenoids. *Int J Pediatr Otorhinolaryngol*, Vol.73, No.12, (December 2009), pp. 1650-2

Alvarez, R.J. & Liu, N.J. (1997). Pediatric ethmoid mucoceles in cystic fibrosis: long-term follow-up of reported cases. *Ear Nose throat J*, Vol.76, No.8, (August 1997), pp. 538-9, pp. 543-6

Arrué, P.; Kany, M.T.; Serrano, E.; Lacroix, F.; Percodani, J.; Yardeni, E.; Pessey, J.J. & Manelfe, C. (1998). Mucoceles of the paranasal sinuses: uncommon location. *J Laryngol Otol*, Vol.112, No.9, (September 1998), pp. 840-4

Avery, G.; Tang, R.A. & Close, L.G. (1983). Ophthalmic manifestations of mucoceles. *Ann Ophthalmol*, Vol.15, No. 8, (August 1983), pp. 734-7

Aydil, U.; Karadeniz H. & Sahin C. (2008). Choanal polyp originated from the inferior nasal concha. *Eur Arch Otorhinolaryngol*, Vol.265, No.4, (April 2008), pp. 477-479

Bachmann, G.; Nekic, M. & Michel, O. (2000). Clinical experience with beta-trace protein as a marker for cerebrospinal fluid. *Ann Otol Rhinol Laryngol*, Vol.109, No.12 Pt 1, (December 2000), pp. 1099-102

Basak, S.; Karaman, C.Z.; Akdilli A. & Metin K.K. (1998). Surgical approaches to antrochoanal polyps in children. *Int J Pediatr Otorhinolaryngol*, Vol.46, No.3, (December 1998), pp. 197-205

Beckhardt, R.N.; Setzen M. & Carras R. (1991). Primary spontaneous cerebrospinal fluid rhinorrhea. *Otolaryngol Head Neck Surg*, Vol.104, No.4, (April 1991), pp. 425-432

Beham, A.; Kainz, J.; Stammberger, H.; Auböck, L. &. Beham-Schmid, C. (1997). Immunohistochemical and electron microscopical characterization of stromal cells in nasopharyngeal angiofibromas. *Eur Arch Otorhinolaryngol*, Vol.254, No.4, (April 1997), pp. 196-9

Beham, A.; Beham-Schmid, C.; Regauer, S.; Auböck, L. & Stammberger, H. (2000). Nasopharyngeal angiofibroma: true neoplasm or vascular malformation? *Adv Anat Pathol*, Vol.7, No.1, (January 2000), pp. 36-46

Berg, O.; Carnfelt, C.; Silfversward C. & Sobin A. (1988). Origin of the choanal polyp. *Arch Otolaryngol Head Neck Surg*, Vol.114, No. 11, (November 1988), pp. 1270-1

Berlucchi, M.; Staurenghi, G.; Rossi Brunori, P.; Tomenzoli, D. & Nicolai, P. (2003). Transnasal endoscopic dacryocystorhinostomy for the treatment of lacrimal pathway stenoses in pediatric patients. *Int J Pediatr Otorhinolaryngol*, Vol.67, No.10, (October 2003), pp. 1069-74

Berlucchi, M.; Salsi, D.; Valetti, L.; Parrinello, G. & Nicolai P. (2007). The role of mometasone furoate aqueous nasal spray in the treatment of adenoid hypertrophy in the pediatric age: preliminary results of a prospective randomized study. *Pediatrics*, Vol.119, No. 6, (June 2007), pp. e1392-7

Berlucchi, M.; Maroldi, R.; Aga, A.; Grazzani, L. & Padoan, R. (2010). Ethmoid mucocele: a new feature of primary ciliary dyskineesia. *Pediatr Pulmonol*, Vol.45, No. 2, (February 2010), pp. 197-201

Berlucchi, M.; Pedruzzi, B. & Farina, D. (2010). Radiology quiz case 2. Lobular capillary hemangioma (LCH). *Arch Otolaryngol Head Neck Surg*, Vol.136, No. 11, (November 2010), pp. 1141, 1143

Bothwell, M.R.; Piccirillo, J.F.; Lusk, R.P. & Ridenour B.D. (2002). Long-term outcome of facial growth after functional endoscopic sinus surgery. *Otolaryngol Head Neck Surg*, Vol.126, No.6, (June 2002), pp. 628-34

Bradley, P.J. & Singh S.D. (1982). Congenital nasal masses: diagnosis and management. *Clin Otolaryngol Allied Sci*, Vol.7, No.2, (April 1982), pp. 87-97

Busaba, N.Y. & Salman, S.D. (1999). Maxillary sinus mucoceles: clinical presentation and long-term results of endoscopic surgical treatment. *Laryngoscope*, Vol.109, No.9, (September 1999), pp. 1446-9

Cassano, P.; Gelardi, M.; Cassano, M.; Fiorella, M.C. & Fiorella R. (2003) Adenoid tissue rhinopharyngeal obstruction grading based on fibroendoscopic findings: a novel approach to therapeutic management. *Int J Ped Otorhinolaryngol*, Vol.61, No.12, (December 2003), pp. 1303-9

Caylakli, F.; Yavuz, H.; Cagici, A.C. & Ozluoglu L.N. (2006). Endoscopic sinus surgery for maxillary sinus mucoceles. *Head Face Med*, Vol.6, No.2, (September 2006), pp. 29

Cingi, C.; Ure, B.; Cakli, H. & Ozudogru E. (2010). Microdebrider-assisted versus radiofrequency-assisted inferior turbinoplasty: a prospective study with objective and subjective outcome measures. *Acta Otorhinolaryngol Ital*, Vol.30, No.3, (June 2010), pp. 138-43

Clarós, P.; Bandos, R.; Clarós, A. Jr; Gilea, I.; Clarós, A. & Real, M. (1998). Nasal gliomas: main features, management and report of five cases. *Int J Pediatr Otorhinolaryngol*, Vol.46, No.1-2, (November 1998), pp. 15-20

Clement, P.A.R. (2008). Rhinosinusitis in children. In: *Pediatric ENT*, J.M. Graham; G.K. Scadding & P.D. Bull, (Eds.), 307-25, Springer, Berlin, Germany

Curtin, H.D. & Rabinov J.D. (1998). Extension to the orbit from paraorbital disease. The sinuses. *Radiol Clin North Am*, Vol.36, No.6, (November 1998), pp. 1201-13

Dabholkar, J.P.; Sathe N.U. & Patole A.D. (2004). Nasal Glioma – A diagnostic challenge. Ind J Otolaryngol Head Neck Surg, Vol.56, No.1, (January 2004), pp. 27-28

De Vuysere S.; Hermans R. & Marchal G. Sinochoanal polyp and its variant, the angiomatous polyp: MRI findings. *Eur Radiol*, Vol.11, No.1, pp. 55-8

Dimov, P.; Rouev, P.; Tenev, K.; Krosneva, R. & Valkanov, P. (2001). Endoscopic surgery for the removal of a nasal glioma: case report. *Otolaryngol Head Neck Surg* Vol.124, No.6, (June 2001), pp. 690

Dunham, M.E. & Miller R.P. (1992). Bilateral choanal atresia associated with malformation of the anterior skull base: embryogenesis and clinical implications. *Ann Otol Rhinol Laryngol*, Vol.101, No.11, (November 1992), pp. 916-9

Durmaz, A.; Tosun, F.; Yldrm, N.; Sahan, M.; Kvrakdal, C. & Gerek M. Transnasal andoscopic repair of choanal atresia: results of 13 cases and meta-analysis. *J Craniofac Surg*, Vol.19, No.5, (September 2008), pp. 1270-4

el-Sayed, Y. & al-Serhani A. (1997). Lobular capillary haemangioma (pyogenic granuloma) of the nose. *J Laryngol Otol*, Vol.111, No.10, (October 1997), pp. 941-5

Fitzpatrick, E. & Miller R.H. (1996). Congenital midline nasal masses: dermoids, gliomas, and encephaloceles. *J La State Med Soc*, Vol.148, No.3, (March 1996), pp. 93-6

Fokkens, W.; Lund, V.; Mullol, J. & European Position Paper on Rhinosinusistis and Nasal Polyps group. (2007). European position paper on rhinosinusistis and nasal polyps 2007. Rhinol Suppl 20, pp.1-136

Frosini, P.; Picarella, G. & De Campora E. (2009). Antrochoanal polyp: analysis of 200 cases. *Acta Otorhinolaryngol Ital*, Vol.29, No.1, (February 2009), pp. 21-6

Guttenplan, M.D. & Wetmore, R.F. (1989). Paranasal sinus mucocele in cystic fibrosis. *Clin Pediatr* (Phila), Vol.28, No.9, (September 1989), pp. 429-30

Han, M.H.; Chang, K.H.; Lee, C.H.; Na, D.G.; Yeon K.M. & Han M.C. (1995). Cystic expansile masses of the maxilla: differential diagnosis with CT and MR. *AJNR Am J Neuroradiol*, Vol.16, No.2, (February 1995), pp. 333-8

Harley, E.H. (1991). Pediatric congenital nasal masses. *Ear Nose Throat J*, Vol.70,No.1, (January 1991), pp. 28-32

Hayasaka, S.; Shibasaki, H.; Sekimoto, M.; Setogawa, T. & Wakutani, T. (1991). Ophthalmic complications in patients with paranasal sinus mucopyoceles. *Ophthalmologica*, Vol.203, No.2, pp. 57-63

Hengerer, A.S. & Newburg J.A. (1990). Congenital malformations of the nose and paranasal sinuses. In: *Pediatric Otolaryngology*, 2nd edition, C.D. Bluestone; S.E. Stool & M.D. Scheetz, (Eds.),718-28, W.B. Saunders Company, Philadelphia, U.S.A.

Hoeger PH, Schaefer H, Ussmueller J, Helmke K. Nasal glioma presenting as capillary haemangioma. Eur J Pediatr 2001;160: 84-7

Hoving, E.W. (2000). Nasal Encephaloceles. *Child's Nerv Syst*, Vol.16, pp. 702–6

Jayaraj, S.M.; Patel, S.K.; Ghufoor, K. & Frosh, A.C. (1999). Mucoceles of the maxillary sinus. *Int J Clin Pract*, Vol.53, No.5, (July-August 1999), pp. 391-3

Jyonouchi, S.; McDonald –Mc-Ginn, D.M.; Bale, S.; Zackai, E.H. & Sullivan, K.E. (2009). CHARGE (coloboma, heart defect, atresia choanae, retarded growth and development, genital hypoplasia, ear anomalies/deafness) syndrome and chromosome 22q11.2 deletion syndrome: a comparison of immunologic and nonimmunologic phenotypic features. *Pediatrics*, Vol.123, No.5, (May 2009), pp. e871-7

Joe, S.A.; Bolger, W.E.; & Kennedy, D.W. (2001). Nasal endoscopy: diagnosis and staging of inflammatory sinus disease, In: *Diseases of the sinuses. Diagnosis and management*, D.W. Kennedy; W.E. Bolger & S.J. Zinreich, (Eds.), 119-128, B.C. Decker Inc, London, England

Johnson, J.T. & Ferguson, B.J. (1998). Infection. In: *Otolaryngology, Head and Neck Surgery*, 3rd edition, C.W. Cummings; J.M. Fredrickson, L.A. Harker; C.J. Krause; D.E. Schuller; M.A. Richardson, (Eds.), 1115-6, Mosby, St. Louis, U.S.A.

Keller, J.L. & Kacker, A. (2000). Choanal atresia, CHARGE association, and congenital nasal stenosis. *Otolaryngol Clin North Am*, Vol.33, No.6, (December 2000), pp. 1343-51

Kennard, C.D. & Rasmussen J.E. (1990). Congenital midline nasal masses: diagnosis and management. *J Dermatol Surg Oncol*, Vol.16, No.11, (November 1990), pp. 1025-36

Kennedy, D.W. (1985). Functional endoscopic sinus surgery. Technique. *Arch Otolaryngol*, Vol.111, No.10, (October 1985), pp. 643-9

Kennedy, D.W. & Senior B.A. (1997). Endoscopic sinus surgery. A review. *Otolaryngol Clin North Am*, Vol.30, No.3, (June 1997), pp. 313-30

Kwok, J.; Leung, MK. & Koltai, P. (2007). Congenital inferior turbinate hypertrophy: an unsual cause of neonatal nasal obstruction. *Int J Pediatr Otorhinolaryngol Extra*, Vol.2, No.1, (March 2007), pp. 26-30

Kosko, J.R.; Hall, B.E. & Tunkel, D.E. (1996). Acquired maxillary sinus hypoplasia: a consequence of endoscopic sinus surgery? *Laryngoscope*, Vol.106 No.10, (October 1996), pp. 1210-3

Lello, G.E.; Sparrow, O.C. & Gopal, R. (1989). The surgical correction of fronto-ethmoidal meningo-encephaloceles. *J Craniomaxillofac Surg* Vol.17, No.7, (October 1989), pp. 293-8

Lieser, J.D. & Derkay, C.S. (2005). Pediatric sinusitis: when do we operate? *Curr Opin Otolaryngol Head Neck Surg*, Vol.13,No.1, (February 2005), pp. 60-6.

Lloyd, G.; Lund, V.J.; Savy L. & Howard D. (2000). Optimum imaging for mucoceles. *J Laryngol Otol*, Vol.114, No.3, (March 2000), pp. 233–6

Lloyd, K.M.; Del Gaudio, J.M. & Hudgins, P.A. (2008). Imaging of skull base cerebrospinal fluid leaks in adults. *Radiology*, Vol.248, No.3, (September 2008), pp. 725-36

Lowe, L.H.; Booth, T.N.; Joglar, J.M. & Rollins, N.K. (2000). Midface anomalies in children. *Radiographics*, Vol.20, No.5, (September-October 2000), pp. 907-22

Lund, V.J. Extended applications of endoscopic sinus surgery — the territorial imperative. *J Laryngol Otol* Vol.111, No.4, (April 1997), pp. 313-5

Lusk, R.P. & Muntz, H. (1990). Endocopic sinus surgery in children with chronic sinusitis: a pilot study. *Laryngoscope*, Vol.100, No.6, (June 1990), pp. ,654-8

Lusk, R.P. (1992). *Pediatric sinusitis*. Raven, New York, U.S.A.

Lusk, R.P. & Stankiewicz, J.A. (1997). Pediatric rhinosinusitis. *Otolaryngol Head Neck Surg*, Vol.117,No.2, (September 1997), pp. S53-S57

Ma, K.H. & Keung, K.L. (2006). Nasal glioma. *Hong Kong Med J*, Vol.12, No.6, (December 2006), pp. 477-9

Mahapatra, A.K. & Suri, A. (2002). Anterior Encephaloceles: a study of 92 Cases. *Pediatr Neurosurg*, Vol.36, No.3, (March 2002), pp. 113–8

Mahapatra, A.K. & Agrawal D. (2006). Anterior encephaloceles: a series of 103 cases over 32 years. *J Clin Neurosci*, Vol.13, No.5, (June 2006), pp. 536–9

Marks, S.C.; Latoni J.D. & Mathog R.H. (1997). Mucoceles of the maxillary sinus. *Otolaryngol Head Neck Surg*, Vol.117, No.1, (july 1997), pp. 18-21

Maroldi, R.; Berlucchi, M.; Farina, D.; Tomenzoli, D.; Borghesi, A. & Pianta, L. Benign neoplasms and tumor-like lesions. In: *Imaging in treatment planning for sinonasal diseases*, R. Maroldi & P. Nicolai, (Eds.), 107-158, Springer, Berlin, Germany

Martin, R.J.; Jackman, D.S.; Philbert, R.F. & McCoy J.M. (2000). Massive proptosis of the globe. *J Oral Maxillofac Surg*, Vol.58, No.7, (July 2000), pp. 794-9

Mc Carty, J.G.; Thorne, C.H.M.; Wood-Smith D. (1990). Principles of craniofacial surgery: Orbital hypertelorism. In: *Plastic Surgery*, J.G. Mc Carty, (Ed.), 2974-3012, WB Saunders Company, Philadelphia, U.S.A.

Messerklinger, W. (1966). On the drainage of the human paranasal sinuses under normal and pathological conditions. 1. *Monatsschr Ohrenheilkd Laryngorhinol,* Vol.100, pp. 56-68

Messerklinger, W. (1967). On the drainage of the human paranasal sinuses under normal and pathological conditions. 2. The frontal sinus and its evacuation system. *Monatsschr Ohrenheilkd Laryngorhinol,* Vol.101, pp. 313-26

Messerklinger, W. (1978). *Endoscopy of the nose.* Urban and Schwarzenberg, Munchen, Germany

Moriyama, H.; Hesaka, H.; Tachibana, T. & Honda, Y. (1992). Mucoceles of ethmoid and sphenoid sinus with visual disturbance. *Arch Otolaryngol Head Neck Surg,* Vol.118, No.2, (February 1992), pp. 142-6

Morris, W.M.; Losken, H.W. & le Roux P.A. (1989). Spheno-maxillary meningo-encephalocele. A case report. J Craniomaxillofac Surg Vol.17, No.8, (November 1989), pp. 359-62

Nachtigal, D.; Frenkiel, S.; Yoskovitch, A. & Mohr, G. (1999). Endoscopic repair of cerebrospinal fluid rhinorrhea: is it the treatment of choice? *J Otolaryngol,* Vol.28, No.3, (January 1999), pp. 129–33

Naidich, T.P.; Altman N.R.; Braffman, B.H.; McLone, D.G. & Zimmerman, R.A. (1992). Cephaloceles and related malformations. *AJNR Am J Neuroradiol,* Vol.13, No2, (March-April 1992), pp. 655–90

Nicolai, P.; Berlucchi, M.; Tomenzoli, D.; Cappiello, J.; Trimarchi, M.; Maroldi, R.; Battaglia, G. & Antonelli, A.R. (2003) Endoscopic surgery for juvenile angiofibroma: when and how. *Laryngoscope,* Vol.113,No.5, (May 2003), pp. 775-82

Nicolai, P.; Lombardi, D.; Tomenzoli, D.; Villaret, A.B.; Piccioni, M.; Mensi, M. & Maroldi, R. (2009). Fungus ball of the paranasal sinuses: experience in 160 patients treated with endoscopy surgery. *Laryngoscope,* Vol.119, No.11, (November 2009), pp. 2275-9

Nicolai, P.; Villaret, A.B.; Farina, D., Nadeau, S.; Yakirevitch, A.; Berlucchi, M. & Galtelli, C. (2010). Endoscopic surgery for juvenile angiofibroma: a critical review of indications after 46 cases. *Am J Rhinol Allergy* Vol.24, No.2, (March 2010), pp. e67-72

Nicolai, P.; Castelnuovo, P. & Bolzoni Villaret A. (2011). Endoscopic resection of sinonasal malignancies. *Curr Oncol Rep* Vol.13, No.2, (April 2011), pp. 138-144

Nicollas, R.; Facon, F.; Sudre-Levillain, I.; Forman, C.; Roman, S. & Triglia J.M. (2006). Pediatric paranasal sinus mucoceles: etiologic factors, management, and outcome. *Int J Pediatr Otorhinolaryngol,* Vol.70, No.5, (May 2006), pp. 905-8

Nuss, D.W. & Costantino P.D. (1995). Diagnosis and Management of Cerebrospinal Fluid Leaks. In: *Highlights of the Instructional Courses of the American Academy of Otolaryngology-Head and Neck Surgery.* F.E. Lucente, (Ed.), Volume 8, Mosby-Yearbook Publishers, St. Louis, U.S.A.

Ohta, N.; Ito, T.; Sasaki, A. & Aoyagi, M. (2010). Endoscopic treatment of intranasal glioma in an infant presenting with dyspnea. *Auris Nasus Larynx,* Vol.37, No.3, (June 2010), pp. 373-6

Olze, H.; Matthias, C. & Degenhardt, P. (2006), Paediatric paranasal sinus mucoceles. *Eur J Pediatr Surg,* Vol.16, No.3, (June 2006), pp. 192-6.

Ommaya, A.K. (1976). Spinal fluid fistulae. *Clin Neurosurg*, Vol. 23, (1976), pp. 363-92

Orvidas, L.J.; Beatty, C.W. & Weaver, A.L. (2001). Antrochoanal polyps in children. *Am J Rhinol*, Vol.15, No.5, (September-October 2001), pp. 321-5

Ozcan, C.; Apa, D.D. & Görür, K. (2004). Pediatric lobular capillary hemangioma of the nasal cavity. *Eur Arch Otorhinolaryngol*, Vol.261, No.8, (September 2004), pp. 449-51

Ozdek, A.; Samim, E.; Bayiz, U.; Meral, I.; Safak, M.A. & Oguz, H. (2002). Antrochoanal polyps in children. *Int J Pediatr Otorhinolaryngol*, Vol.65, No.3, (September 2002), pp. 213-8

Palfyn J. Anatomie chirurgicale. Paris, 1753.

Pakkasjärvi, N.; Salminen, P.; Kalajoki-Helmiö, T.; Rintala, R. & Pitkäranta, A. (2008). Respiratory distress secondary to nasopharyngeal glial heterotopia. *Eur J Pediatr Surg*, Vol.18, No.2, (August 2008), pp. 117-8

Pelikan, Z. (2009). Role of nasal allergy in chronic secretory otitis media. *Curr Allergy Asthma Rep*, Vol.9, No.2, (March 2009), pp. 107-13

Pianta, L.; Pinelli, L.; Nicolai, P. & Maroldi, R. Cerebrospinal fluid leak, meningocele and meningoencephalocele. In: *Imaging in treatment planning for sinonasal diseases*, R. Maroldi & P. Nicolai, (Eds.), 93-106, Springer, Berlin, Germany

Presutti, L.; Mattioli, F.; Villari, D.; Marchioni, D. & Alicandri-Ciufelli, M. (2009). Transnasal endoscopic treatment of cerebrospinal fluid leak: 17 years' experience. *Acta Otorhinolaryngol Ital*, Vol.29, No.4, (August 2009), pp. 191-6

Pruna, X.; Ibanez, J.M.; Serres, X.; Garriga, V; Barber, I. & Vera, J. (2000) Antrochoanal polyps in children: CT findings and differential diagnosis. *Eur Radiol*, Vol.10, No.5, (2000), pp. 849-51

Puppala, B.; Mangurten, H.H.; McFadden, J.; Lygizos, N.; Taxy, J. & Pellettiere, E. (1990). Nasal glioma presenting as neonatal respiratory distress. Definition of the tumor mass by MRI. *Clin Pediatr (Phil)*, Vol.29, No.1, (January 1990), pp. 49-52

Puxeddu, R.; Berlucchi, M.; Ledda, G.P.; Parodo, G.; Farina, D. & Nicolai, P. (2006). Lobular capillary hemangioma of the nasal cavity: a retrospective study on 40 patients. *Am J Rhinol*, Vol.20, No.4, (July-August 2006), pp. 480-4

Rahbar, R.; Resto, V.A.; Robson, C.D.; Perez-Atayde, A.R.; Goumnerova, L.C.; McGill, T.J. & Healy, G.B. (2003). Nasal glioma and encephalocele: diagnosis and management. *Laryngoscope*, Vol.113, No.12, (December 2003), pp. 2069-77

Samadi, D.S.; Shah, U.K.; Handler, S.D. (2003). Choanal atresia: a twenty-year review of medical comorbidities and surgical outcomes. *Laryngoscope*, Vol.113, No.2, (February 2003), pp. 254-8.

Samii, M. & Draf, W. (1989). Surgery of malformations of the anterior skull base. In: *Surgery of the Skull Base*, M. Samii & W. Draf (Eds), 114-26, Springer-Verlag, Berlin, Germany

Schlosser, R.J. & Bolger, W.E. (2002). Nasal cerebrospinal fluid leaks. *J Otolaryngol*, Vol.31, Suppl.1, (August 2002), pp. S28–S37

Schramm, V.L. Jr. & Effron, M.Z. (1980). Nasal polyps in children. *Larygoscope*, Vol.90, No.9, (September 1980), pp. 1488-95

Schweinfurth, J.M. (2002). Image guidance-assisted repair of bilateral choanal atresia. *Laryngoscope*, Vol.112, No.11, (November 2002), pp. 2096-8

Senior, B.; Wirtschafter, A.; Mai, C.; Becker, C. & Belenky,W. (2000). Quantitative impact of pediatric sinus surgery on facial growth. *Laryngoscope*, Vol.110, No.11, (November 2000), pp. 1866-70

Składzień, J.; Litwin, J.A.; Nowogrodzka-Zagórska, M. & Wierzchowski, W. (2001). Morphological and clinical characteristics of antrochoanal polyps: comparison with chronic inflammation-associated polyps of the maxillary sinus. *Auris Nasus Larynx*, Vol.28, No.2, (April 2001), pp. 137-41

Som, P.M. & Brandwein, M. (1996). Sinonasal cavities. Inflammatory disease, tumors, fractures, and postoperative findings. In: *Head and Neck Imaging*, P.M. Som & H.D. Curtin, (Eds.), 3rd edition, 126–85, Mosby, St. Louis, U.S.A.

Stammberger, H. (1999). 2. Surgical treatment of nasal polyps: past, present and future. *Allergy*, Vol.54, Suppl.53, (1999), pp. 7-11

Suwanwela, C. & Suwanwela, N. (1972). A morphological classification of sincipital encephalomeningocele. *J Neusurg*, Vol.36, No.2, (February 1972), pp. 201-11

Teissier, N.; Kaguelidou, F.; Couloigner, V.; Francois, M. & Van Den Abbeele, T. (2008). Predictive factors for success after transnasal endoscopic treatment of coanal atresia. *Arch Otolaryngol Head Neck Surg*, Vol.134, No.1, (January 2008), pp. 57-61

Thomé, D.C.; Voegels, R.L.; Cataldo de la Cortina, R.A. & Butugan, O. (2000). Bilateral ethmoidal mucocele in cystic fibrosis: report of a case. *Int J Pediatr Otorhinolaryngol*, Vol.55, No.2, (September 2000), pp. 143-8

Triglia, J.M. & Nicollas, R. (1997). Nasal and sinus polyposis in children. *Laryngoscope*, Vol.107, No.7, (July 1997), pp. 963-6

Tseng, C.C.; Ho, C.Y. & Kao, S.C. (2005). Ophthalmic manifestations of paranasal sinus mucoceles. *J Chin Med Assoc*, Vol.68, No.6, (June 2005), pp. 260-4.

Uzunlar, A.K.; Osma, U.; Yilmaz, F. & Topcu, U. (2001). Nasal glioma: report of two cases. *Turk J Med Sci*, Vol.31, pp. 87-90

Van Peteghem, A. & Clement, P.A. (2006). Influence of extensive functional endoscopic sinus surgery (FESS) on facial growth in children with cystic fibrosis. Comparison of 10 cephalometric parameters of the midface for three study groups. *Int J Pediatr Otorhinolaryngol*, Vol.70, No.8, (August 2006), pp. 1407-13

Varghese, L.; John, M. & Kurien, M. (2004). Bilateral asymmetric mucoceles of the paranasal sinuses: a first case report. *Ear Nose Throat J*, Vol.83, No.12, (December 2004), pp. 834-5

Vatansever, U.; Duran, R.; Acunas, B.; Koten, M. & Adali, M.K. (2005). Bilateral choanal atresia in premature monozygotic twins. *J Perinatol*, Vol.25, No.12, (December 2005), pp. 800-2

Vuckovic, N.; Vuckovic, D.; Dankuc, D. & Jovancevic, L. (2006). Nasal glioma. *Arch Oncol*, Vol.14, No.1-2, (June 2006), pp. 57-9

Wolf, C.; Greistorfer, K. & Jebeles, J.A. (1995). The endoscopic endonasal surgical technique in the treatment of chronic recurring sinusitis in children. *Rhinology*, Vol.33, No.2, (June 1995), pp. 97-103

Wong, R.K. & VanderVeen, D.K. (2008). Presentation and management of congenital dacryocystocele. *Pediatrics*, Vol.122, No.5, (November 2008), pp. e1108-12.

Woodworth, B.A.; Schlosser, R.J.; Faust, R.A. & Bolger, W.E. (2004). Evolutions in the management of congenital intranasal skull base defects. *Arch Otolaryngol Head Neck Surg*, Vol.130, No.11, (November 2004), pp. 1283-88

Yaman, H.; Yilmaz, S.; Karali, E.; Guclu, E. & Ozturk, O. (2010). Evaluation and management of antrochoanal polyps. *Clin Exp Otorhinolaryngol*, Vol.3, No.2, (June 2010), pp. 110-4

Yerkes, S.A.; Thompson D.H. & Fisher, W.S. (1992). Spontaneous cerebrospinal fluid rhinorrhea. *Ear Nose Throat J, Vol.* 71, No.7, (July 1992), pp 318–20

7

Endoscopy in the Evaluation and Management of the Pediatric Airway

Kris R. Jatana[1] and Jeffrey C. Rastatter[2]
[1]Nationwide Children's Hospital and The Ohio State University Columbus, Ohio
[2]Children's Memorial Hospital and Northwestern University Chicago, Illinois
USA

1. Introduction

The airway starts at the anterior nasal vestibule and ends at the lung parenchyma. This includes the nasal cavity, nasopharynx, oral cavity, oropharynx, larynx, hypopharynx, trachea, and bronchi. When evaluating a child with noisy breathing, it is important to assess the airway in a systematic manner.

A thorough history is important. This includes assessment of the severity or progression of symptoms, and whether the symptoms are worse with feeding or increased exertion. The severity determines the urgency of complete evaluation. Apparent life-threatening events (ALTE) warrant prompt multidisciplinary evaluation (McMurray, 1997).

Inspiratory stridor generally originates from the larynx, while expiratory stridor from the trachea or bronchi. Stridor that is biphasic (both inspiratory and expiratory) typically indicates a fixed obstructive lesion is present. Depending on symptomatology, the addition of endoscopic evaluation of the airway to the basic physical examination can be extremely beneficial. A definitive diagnosis is critical to proper treatment intervention.

2. Types of endoscopy

Endoscopic evaluation of the pediatric airway can be accomplished with both rigid and flexible endoscopes. It can be done awake in the office or under general anesthesia. In the office, awake flexible endoscopic examination of the nasal cavity, nasopharynx, oropharynx, hypopharynx, and larynx can be performed. Rigid endoscopy, using various sizes and degrees of scopes, is used to evaluate the nasal cavity and nasopharynx. Transoral rigid endoscopy with an angled scope to evaluate the oropharynx, hypopharyx, or larynx is not well-tolerated in children. Awake flexible fiberoptic endoscopy allows for full assessment of the upper airway to the level of the true vocal cords. An advantage to awake exanimation is that direct visualization of the airway can be correlated with the noisy breathing of the child, helping to identify the cause. Vocal cord function is best assessed using awake flexible fiberoptic laryngoscopy. In the past, awake evaluation of the upper airway in children was limited to the level of the true vocal cords, however there is some evidence that flexible fiberoptic laryngoscopy with tracheoscopy can be performed in the office setting without complications (Hartzell, 2010). Due to potential risk of laryngospasm and airway compromise, such evaluation is generally done in the operating room. Under general anesthesia, the assessment of the airway is best for static lesions, however, if the patient can be kept breathing spontaneously, a more dynamic assessment of the lower airways (trachea and bronchi) can be performed. A rigid bronchoscope allows for ventilation (providing adequate time for complete inspection) as well as visualization of the segmental bronchi. While some advocate using a telescope alone to evaluate the trachea and proximal main bronchus, it is difficult to examine the distal portions of each main bronchus and the segmental bronchi.

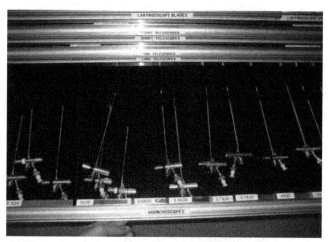

Fig. 1. Equipment

An operating room with systematic organization of various sizes of rigid bronchoscopes, telescopes, laryngoscopes, and flexible fiberoptic scopes.

3. Abnormalities of the nasal cavity

3.1 Nasal vestibular stenosis and pyriform aperature stenosis

Nasal vestibular stenosis results from disruption of the vestibular lining with proliferation of granulation and fibrous tissue. It has occurred in association with nasal CPAP use (Jatana 2008,2010), prior nasal surgical procedures, nasal packing (Karen 2000), excessive cautery for epistaxis (Bajaj, 1969), birth trauma (Jablon, 1997), and flash burn injury (Salvado, 2008). Anterior nasal endoscopy may be required to look for vestibular stenosis, and it can be significant in a neonate who is an obligate nasal breather.

Congenital nasal pyriform aperature stenosis, is a different entity causing a narrowing at the level of the pyriform aperature (Ramadan, 1995).

3.2 Nasal septal deviation

This is a common finding on endoscopy of the nasal cavity. The nasal septum is composed of cartilage and bone, and deformities can contribute to nasal obstruction. This can be developmental or acquired due to nasal trauma. A statistically significant higher incidence of nasal septal deformities has been shown with a history of nasal injury (Zielnik-Jurkiewicz, 2006)

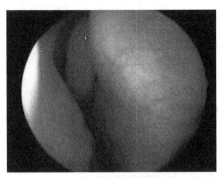

Fig. 2. Nasal septal deviation

Nasal endoscopy using a 0 degree endoscope in the right nasal cavity, showing a nasal septal deformity to the right compromising the nasal airway.

3.3 Nasal polyposis

Nasal endoscopy can be useful in the diagnosis of nasal polyps which generally result from chronic inflammation. The development may be related to chronic rhinosinusitis, asthma, allergic rhinitis, or cystic fibrosis (Triglia, 1997). Patients with cystic fibrosis, an autosomal recessive condition, frequently develop chronic rhinosinusitis with or without nasal polyps (Franco, 2009; Weber, 2008). Imaging is critical prior to any surgical intervention as tumors or masses with intracranial extension can be present in the sinonasal cavity of children. Endoscopic sinus surgery can be used to remove polyps as indicated.

3.4 Anterior cranial fossa masses

Dermoid sinus (with/without intracranial extension), encephaloceles, and gliomas are the most common midline nasal masses (Hughes, 1980), and imaging must be performed prior to any surgical intervention. If intracranial extension is not known, there is risk of CSF leak, meningitis, or intracranial injury (Hedlund, 2006). If a skull base defect is present, it may need to be repaired simultaneously which can be done either endoscopically or by craniotomy depending on the size and intracranial extent.

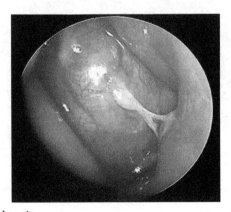

Fig. 3. Cystic mass, nasal cavity

This rare nasal mass, a chondromesencymal hamartoma, is a benign congenital lesion that has known propensity to have intracranial extension. This can mimic the appearance of a meningoencephalocele (Kim 2004).

3.5 Choanal atresia

A failure of the posterior nasal aperature to canalize results in choanal atresia, and this can be unilateral or bilateral. It was first described in 1755 by Roederer and occurs in 1 of 5000-7000 live births. A newborn is an obligate nasal breather. Neonates with bilateral choanal atresia require endotracheal intubation at the time of birth (Deutsch, 1997). It has been shown that 71% of these are mixed (bony and membranous), and 29% are bony atresia (Brown, 1996). Nasal endoscopy can be used to show the atretic plate in the back of the nasal cavity along the nasal floor. In most cases, repair can be successfully performed endoscopically (Hengerer, 2008; Ramsden, 2009).

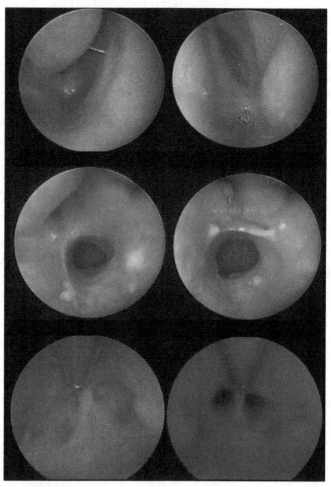

Fig. 4. Bilateral choanal atresia

At the top, a 0 degree endoscope in the nasal cavity of a newborn child who had respiratory distress immediately at birth. Note the blocked choana bilaterally (right & left). The middle image shows the right and left posterior nasal cavity, 2 weeks after endoscopic repair. At the bottom is a view through a 120 degree endoscope with the soft palate retracted anteriorly. Note the posterior choana before (left) and after (right) endoscopic repair.

3.6 Nasal septal perforation

The nasal septum, consisting of both cartilage and bone, divides the left and right nasal cavities. A perforation, or hole, in the septum can cause non-specific symptoms, including epistaxis, obstruction, crusting, whistling, and pain. Causes of perforation include: chronic trauma, piercings, intranasal placement of button batteries, drug use (including cocaine), industrial metal plating solutions, intranasal steroid use, surgical trauma, nasal cautery, Wegener granulomatosis, sarcoidosis, and syphilis (Diamantopoulos, 2001; Lanier, 2009). Some large nasal septal perforations have been repaired using an endoscope-assisted approach (Giacomini, 2011).

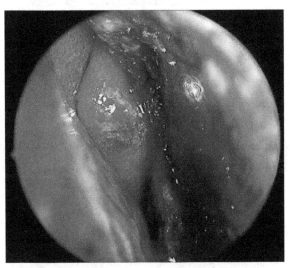

Fig. 5. Right nasal cavity. When placed inside of the body, button batteries need to be removed as soon as possible (emergently), to avoid serious complications.

Note early tissue necrosis (black) after removal of button battery, often resulting in a nasal septal perforation.

4. Abnormalities of the nasopharynx

4.1 Adenoid hypertrophy

The adenoid tissue in the nasopharynx, consists of lymphoid tissue, which is typically small at birth and enlarges to various degrees during early childhood. It often involutes during late childhood. Obstructive adenoid tissue can be related to nasal obstruction symptoms (snoring), eustachian tube dysfunction, and chronic sinusitis. Adenoidectomy is one of the most common surgical procedures done in children.

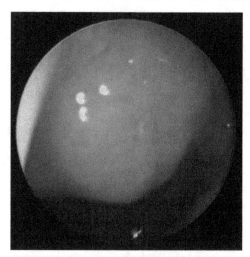

Fig. 6. Adenoid tissue, nasopharynx

The adenoid tissue can be easily visualized transnasally with a 0 degree endoscope, note the moderate obstruction in this patient.

4.2 Meningocele

A meningocele in the nasopharynx must be kept in the differential diagnosis of pediatric nasopharyngeal masses. It has a cystic appearance, originates intracranially from herniation of meninges, and is filled with cerebral spinal fluid (CSF). A congenital defect in the skull base is usually present, and both CT and MRI are critical for surgical planning.

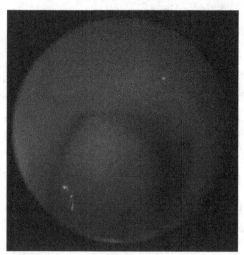

Fig. 7. Cystic mass, nasopharynx

This was a skull base meningocele in a 6 week old child. It was filled with clear fluid (CSF), repair of the skull base defect is necessary to avoid CSF leak and reduce risk of meningitis.

Note the limitation of picture definition and brightness when the surgeon has to use a smaller diameter telescope lens.

4.3 Juvenile Nasopharyngeal Angiofibroma (JNA)

JNA is a benign vascular tumor that arises in the nasopharynx of adolescent males. It often presents with unilateral recurrent epistaxis or nasal obstruction. JNAs originate from the sphenopalatine foramen, commonly extend to the nasal cavity and nasopharynx, and can also extend to the pterygopalatine fossa, infratemporal fossa, orbit, or intracranially. Transnasal rigid or flexible endoscopy typically gives good visualization of the lesion. JNAs can often be removed with minimally invasive endoscopic surgery (Douglas, 2006), while some require traditional open surgical approaches (Bales, 2002).

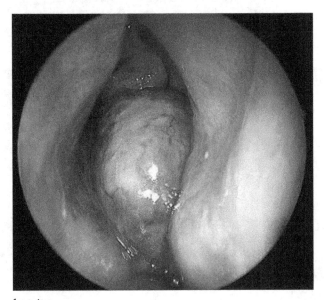

Fig. 8. Right nasal cavity

A JNA originating from the right sphenopalatine foramen, some tumor necrosis is present (white) after pre-resection arterial embolization.

4.4 Nasopharyngeal hamartoma

A hamartoma is a benign, abnormal proliferation of normal tissue. It can be composed of tissue from all 3 germ layers. In the head and neck region they can be found in the oral cavity, nasal cavity, and nasopharynx (Hulsmann, 2009). The overall incidence of nasal hamatomas is 1 in 20,000 to 40,000 live births (Harley, 1991).

5. Abnormalities of the oropharynx

5.1 Lingual Thyroglossal Duct Cyst

Thyroglossal duct cysts (TGDCs) are congenital and can arise at any point along the typical path of the thyroid gland during embryogenesis. Initially formed in the midline base of tongue, the thyroid gland descends to the final location low in the anterior midline of the neck. TGDC is the most common congenital pediatric neck mass (Koeller, 1999). When found in the oropharynx at the base of tongue, these lesions are termed lingual TGDCs. Transnasal flexible fiberoptic laryngoscopy can often visualize these at the tongue base. Endoscopic surgery for removal has also been described (Burkhart, 2009). Proper diagnosis and treatment is important as swelling or growth can lead to airway obstruction (Kuint, 1997; Fu, 2008).

5.2 Vallecular cyst

A vallecular cyst is simple cyst, typically lined with respiratory epithelium and mucous glands, which forms on the lingual surface of the epiglottis (Gutierrez, 1999). They typically present with stridor, feeding problems, and upper airway obstruction (Gluckman, 1992, LaBagnara, 1989). They can be visualized and diagnosed with flexible fiberoptic laryngoscopy. Marsupialization of the cyst is typically curative.

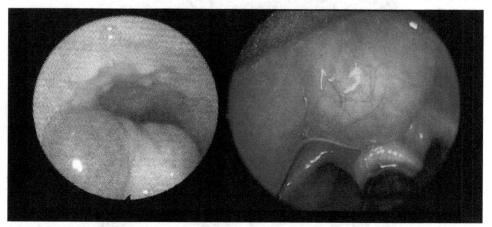

Fig. 9. Vallecular Cyst

On left, using a flexible fiberoptic laryngoscope placed into the nasopharynx (looking down at the tongue base), a large cystic mass originating from vallecula. Posteriorly there is evidence of cobblestoning of the pharyngeal wall. On right a vallecular cyst in a neonate which caused an apparent life-threatening event (ALTE).

6. Abnormalities of the hypopharynx

6.1 Pyriform sinus tracts

Tracts originating from the pyriform sinus within the hypopharynx have also been referred to as third or fourth branchial sinuses, fistulas, or remnants. The vast majority are left-sided, but rarely can occur on the right or be bilateral. These can be the etiology of recurrent neck abscesses or thyroiditis. Treatment options include cautery of the sinus orifice and definitive surgical excision of the tract including thyroid lobectomy. Recently, endoscopic cautery has been advocated as the initial treatment option as it carries less potential morbidity than open excision. (Chen, 2009; Verret, 2004)

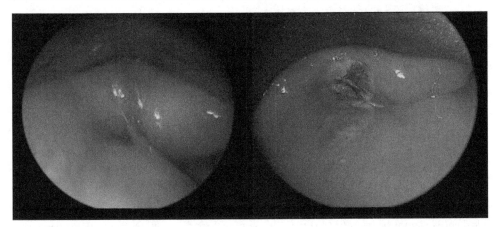

Fig. 10. Pyriform sinus fistula

On the left, note the fistula opening in the left pyriform sinus. On the right, endoscopic cautery was performed using silver nitrate to obliterate the opening which is the source of bacterial contamination of the tract.

7. Abnormalities of the larynx

7.1 Supraglottis and glottis

Flexible fiberoptic laryngoscopy can be used for excellent visualization of the supraglottis and glottis. This is often done initially in the outpatient clinic setting as this procedure is very well tolerated in awake infants and children. Laryngomalacia is the most common congenital laryngeal anomaly causing stridor in infants (Thompson, 2007). Inspiration leads to dynamic collapse of supraglottic structures, the cause of the upper airway obstruction and stridor. Failure of the primitive larynx to recanalize during the tenth week of embryogenesis can lead to laryngeal web formation (McGill, 2000). As they are most

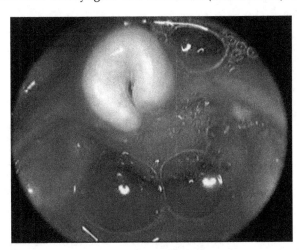

Fig. 11. Laryngomalacia

common at the level of the glottis with variable extension to the subglottis, symptoms include a weak voice and/or upper airway obstruction. Saccular cysts and laryngoceles also are abnormal dilations of the laryngeal saccule that contain either mucoid fluid or air respectively. They can present as swellings in the area of the false vocal fold as seen on flexible fiberoptic laryngoscopy. These relatively rare lesions have been characterized in detail in the literature (Holinger, 1978; DeSanto, 1970). Vocal cord paralysis is best assessed on awake flexible fiberoptic laryngoscopy. Static evaluation of the posterior larynx with a probe is necessary to look for a laryngeal cleft (type I-IV). Children can present with symptoms of stridor, aspiration, and/or respiratory distress (Rahbar 2006). While all type IV clefts require open surgical repair, correction can be done endoscopically in type I-II clefts, and even some type III clefts (Garabedian 2010).

Note the "omega" or "tubular" shaped epiglottis. The aryepiglottic folds are shortened, pulling arytenoids anteriorly. Collapse on inspiration causes stridor and can be directly correlated in the office setting. In severe cases, on awake flexible fiberoptic laryngoscopy the vocal cords cannot be visualized due to this supraglottic obstruction. Supraglottoplasty can be performed in severe cases with failure to thrive or respiratory compromise.

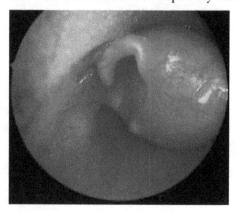

Fig. 12. Right saccular cyst

Note the significant upper airway obstruction that can be present.

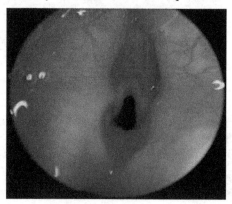

Fig. 13. Glottic web

The vocal cords have limited mobility due to an anterior glottic web. This narrows the glottic airway causing biphasic stridor. Endoscopic surgical repair can be performed.

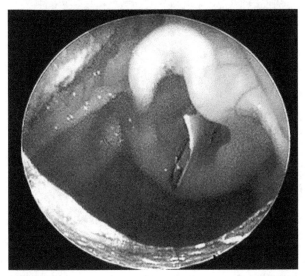

Fig. 14. Glottic foreign body

A pencil shaving lodged in the glottis of a child with severe stridor. This was emergently removed in the operating room.

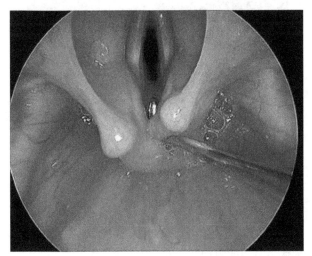

Fig. 15. Normal larynx

A right angle probe can be used to palpate the interarytenoid notch to check for a posterior laryngeal cleft. It is also helpful to palpate the posterior cricoid lamina with a right angle probe to ensure there is no divot or absence of cartilage.

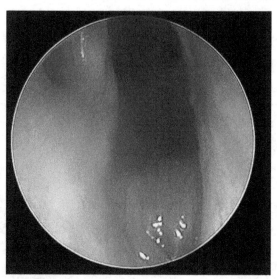

Fig. 16. Type I posterior laryngeal cleft

The interarytenoid notch is below the level of the true vocal cord. With palpation, the cricoids cartilage is intact. Aspiration of thin liquids often can occur, but many infants do well with a thickened diet. If aspiration fails to resolve with time, endoscopic repair can be performed.

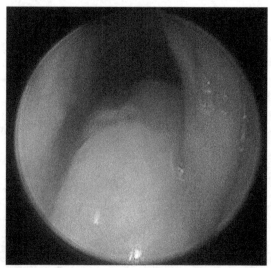

Fig. 17. Type III posterior laryngeal cleft

The cleft extends down through the cricoid cartilage below the vocal cords. With palpation, there is only a cleft of soft tissue posteriorly, no posterior cricoid lamina. It does not enter the thoracic cavity, so is therefore a type III. This cleft is a direct connection between the esophagus and trachea leading to aspiration with feeding.

7.2 The subglottis

The subglottic region is generally difficult to visualize on awake flexible fiberoptic laryngoscopy in the office setting. Subglottic stenosis can be congenital or acquired, and open laryngotracheal reconstruction has been successful (Cotton 2000). Endoscopic management including dilation, laser, mitomycin c, and steroids have also been used (Quensel 2011).

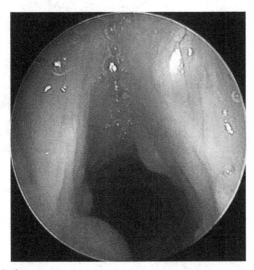

Fig. 18. Glottic and subglottic cysts

Commonly as a result of intubation, sometimes ductal cysts form from occluded submucosal glands. These can be asymptomatic if small.

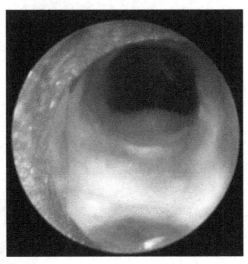

Fig. 19. Intubation injury

Erosion of mucosa overlying posterior cricoid lamina, due to direct pressure from endotracheal tube. Exposed cartilage is seen posteriorly (white). This can lead to subglottic stenosis after intubation.

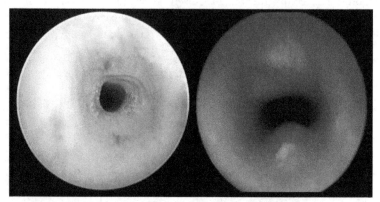

Fig. 20. Congenital subglottic stenosis

Note the narrowing below the vocal cords at the level of the cricoid cartilage and first tracheal ring, Grade III in this patient. This same patient, after a laryngotracheal reconstruction with anterior thyroid ala cartilage graft, the post-operative bronchoscopy shows a well-mucosalized graft.

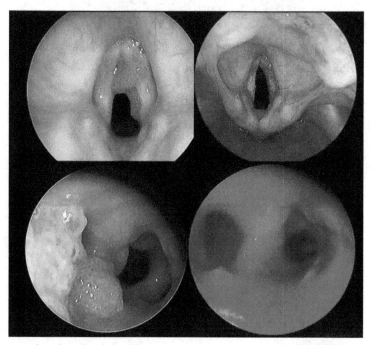

Fig. 21. Laryngeal and tracheal papilloma

Top left: Endoscopic view of the true vocal cords, showing laryngeal papilloma of the right true vocal cord; Top right: After endoscopic removal using microdebrider. Bottom left, tracheal papilloma at the carina; bottom right, after endoscopic surgical removal.

7.3 Recurrent Respiratory Papillomatosis (RRP)

RRP is the most common benign neoplasm of the larynx and the second most common cause of hoarseness in children. It is caused by human papilloma virus and can have either childhood or adult onset. There is no cure for RRP and malignant transformation can rarely occur. Due to location and airway obstruction, surgical debulking is necessary in symptomatic patients. Adjuvant therapies include cidofovir, acyclovir, ribavirin, interferon, photodynamic therapy, indole-3-carbinol, cox-2 inhibitors, and retenoids. A quadravalent HPV vaccine is available and may help reduce the incidence of RRP in the future. (Derkay, 2008). Extra-esophageal reflux has been linked to the disease course in some patients with RRP (McKenna, 2005; Pignatari, 2007).

8. Abnormalities of the tracheobronchial tree

8.1 Tracheobronchomalacia

A condition where there is collapse of the lumen due either intrinsic (primary) or extrinsic factors (secondary). The extraluminal pressure exceeds the intraluminal pressure and can be most significant on expiration. This can cause significant airway obstruction (Austin, 2003; Boogaard 2005). Tracheomalacia is commonly seen in patients with tracheoesophageal fistula.

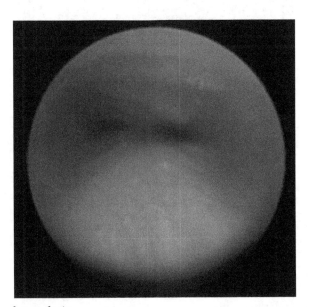

Fig. 22. Severe tracheomalacia

Narrowing of tracheal lumen is seen in a child with tracheoesophageal fistula.

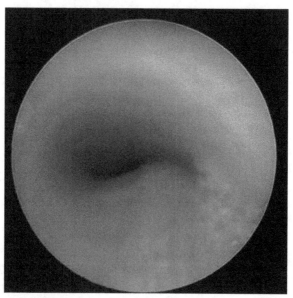

Fig. 23. Severe tracheomalacia

Narrowing of the tracheal lumen is seen with a coin in the esophagus causing external compression of the tracheal airway.

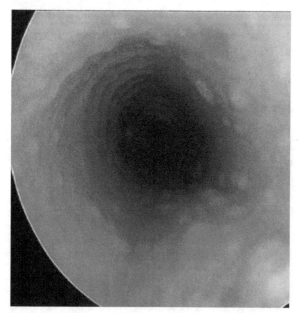

Fig. 24. Chronic follicular tracheitis

Raised mucosal follicles, often seen with acid reflux into the airway.

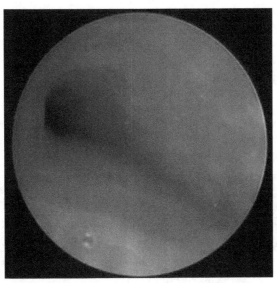

Fig. 25. Bronchomalacia

Narrowing of the left bronchial lumen is seen through a rigid bronchoscope as well as follicular changes of the mucosa.

8.2 Complete tracheal rings

A rare condition characterized by complete cartilaginous rings of the trachea, which can be of short segments or the entire length of the trachea. The surgical management of this condition has evolved over the past two decades (Backer, 2001). Currently, reconstruction methods can include excision of short segments with end-to-end anastomosis and slide tracheoplasty for longer segments (Russell, 2010). A slide tracheoplasty, unless done in a cervical tracheal location, is often done on cardiopulmonary bypass. Often a vascular anomaly, such as pulmonary artery sling is present, and it can be repaired simultaneously (Rutter 2003). Tracheal reconstruction has been successful in even patients with unilateral lung agenesis or severe hypoplasia (Backer, 2009).

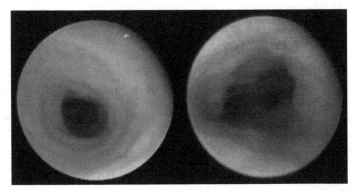

Fig. 26. Complete tracheal rings

Note the concentric complete rings, absent membranous trachea posteriorly, resulting in a distal tracheal stenosis. On the right, the same patient 6 weeks after undergoing a slide tracheoplasty

8.3 Airway hemangioma

A hemangioma is a benign, vascular tumor. Rarely, these arise in the airway and can cause airway obstruction in the first year of life.Treatment options have included endoscopic resection, open resection, systemic or injectable steroids, tracheostomy (to bypass obstruction), interferon, observation (Rahbar, 2004) and more recently, propanolol therapy (Maturo, 2010).

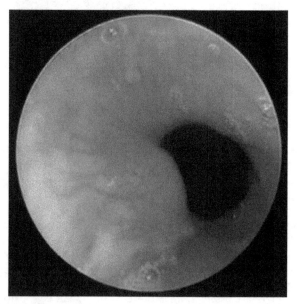

Fig. 27. Tracheal hemangioma

A left-posterior tracheal hemangioma at the level of the 3rd tracheal ring. These are more commonly seen in the subglottis.

8.4 Tracheobronchial foreign body and plastic bronchitis

Bronchial foreign bodies can be life-threatening due to acute airway obstruction. Anatomically, an inhaled foreign body is most likely to enter the right bronchial tree in children of all ages as the proximal right main bronchus is generally steeper and wider than the left (Tahir, 2009). Rigid bronchoscopy is not only diagnostic but also therapeutic using optical forceps to remove foreign bodies under direct visualization. While ventilating the patient through the scope. Communication between the surgeon and anesthesiologist is critical for optimal results (Zur, 2009).

Plastic bronchitis is rare condition where bronchial casts form resulting in life-threatening obstruction. This has been associated with congenital heart disease, particularly after patients undergo a Fontan procedure (Tzifa,2005; Ishman, 2003; Preciado,

2010). Other causes of bronchial casts include cystic fibrosis, asthma, and influenza H1N1 (Terano 2010). The exact etiology for these is unknown, and treatment includes immediate endoscopic removal of the airway obstruction. Various adjuvant therapies including chest physiotherapy, aerosolized urokinase and tissue plasminogen activator, corticosteroids, DNase, and macrolides have been used with limited success (Brogan, 2002; Preciado, 2010)

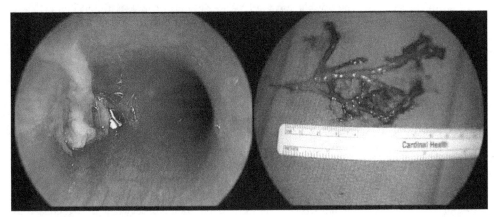

Fig. 28. Plastic bronchitis

Cast formation within the left bronchus before (left) and after (right) endoscopic removal.

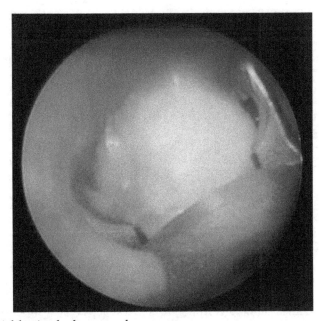

Fig. 29. Bronchial foreign body removal

The optical graspers (telescope with attached camera) through a rigid bronchoscope are used to remove a molar tooth unusually lodged in the the left upper bronchus.

8.5 Vascular rings

A "vascular ring" refers to any anomaly of the aortic arch that leads to compression of the trachea, and/or esophagus. Most children will present early in life with breathing and feeding difficulties. Only the double aortic arch and right aortic arch with left ligament are true complete vascular rings; the innominate artery compression and pulmonary artery sling are incomplete from an anatomical standpoint. Endoscopic evaluation with laryngoscopy and bronchoscopy is helpful to assess the degree of airway compression (Shah, 2007; Russell, 2010).

The double aortic arch occurs when two arches arise at the ascending aorta, pass around both sides of the trachea and esophagus, to join the descending aorta. The right aortic arch occurs when the apex of the arch is to the right side of the trachea; various configurations are possible. Innominate artery compression of the anterior trachea is often due to a more left and posterior origination from the aorta (Russell 2010). If severe, suspension of the innominate artery to the posterior aspect of the sternum has been performed (Moes, 1975). Bronchoscopic evaluation after suspension confirms adequate relief. Pulmonary artery sling occurs when the left pulmonary artery originates from the right pulmonary artery, coursing around the right main bronchus and distal trachea, between the trachea and esophagus, to return to the left side. Pulmonary artery sling is often associated with complete tracheal rings and surgical correction of both can be performed simultaneously (Russell 2010).

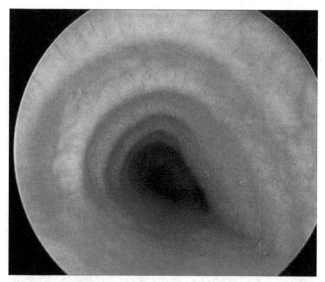

Fig. 30. Tracheomalacia, secondary to vascular ring

A child with a double aortic arch, prior to surgical repair, note the external tracheal compression causing airway obstruction.

8.6 Blunt laryngotracheal trauma

Blunt trauma to the anterior neck can be a life-threatening injury. Significant injury in children is not common as the larynx is higher in location within the neck, and the laryngeal cartilage structures are more flexible than adults. Symptoms can include hoarseness, stridor, respiratory distress, subcutaneous emphysema, dysphagia, neck pain, and hemoptysis. In a stable child with suspected injury, flexible endoscopic evaluation of the larynx can be performed to determine if further surgical intervention would be needed (Gold, 1997). Endotracheal intubation of such cases can be catastrophic resulting in laryngotracheal separation and death (Bernat, 2005). In severe injury, tracheotomy is required for obtaining a stable airway. Children often cannot undergo an awake tracheotomy procedure under local anesthesia, so rigid bronchoscopy using a ventilating scope is critical in securing the airway prior to tracheotomy and open surgical repair.

9. Conclusion

The advancement in endoscopic technology combined with contemporary surgical applications has helped progress the field of diagnostic airway evaluation in children, as well as therapeutic interventions. Certainly, with enhanced visualization, the ability to more safely manage the airway allows for optimal care of children with congenital and acquired anomalies. There is a definite role for endoscopic surgery in pediatric otolaryngology.

10. References

Austin J, Ali T. Tracheomalacia and bronchomalacia in children: pathophysiology, assessment, treatment and anaesthesia management. Paediatr Anaesth 2003;13:3-11.

Backer CL, Kelle AM, Mavroudis C, Rigsby CK, Kaushal S, Holinger LD. Tracheal reconstruction in children with unilateral lung agenesis or severe hypoplasia. Ann Thorac Surg 2009;88:624-30; discussion 30-1.

Backer CL, Mavroudis C, Gerber ME, Holinger LD. Tracheal surgery in children: an 18-year review of four techniques. Eur J Cardiothorac Surg 2001;19:777-84.

Bajaj PS, Bailey BN. Stenosis of the nostrils: a report of three cases. Br J Plast Surg 1969;22:269-73.

Bales C, Kotapka M, Loevner LA, et al. Craniofacial resection of advanced juvenile nasopharyngeal angiofibroma. Arch Otolaryngol Head Neck Surg 2002;128:1071-8.

Bernat RA, Zimmerman JM, Keane WM, Pribitkin EA. Combined laryngotracheal separation and esophageal injury following blunt neck trauma. Facial Plast Surg 2005;21:187-90.

Boogaard R, Huijsmans SH, Pijnenburg MW, Tiddens HA, de Jongste JC, Merkus PJ. Tracheomalacia and bronchomalacia in children: incidence and patient characteristics. Chest 2005;128:3391-7.

Brogan TV, Finn LS, Pyskaty DJ, Jr., et al. Plastic bronchitis in children: a case series and review of the medical literature. Pediatr Pulmonol 2002;34:482-7.

Brown OE, Pownell P, Manning SC. Choanal atresia: a new anatomic classification and clinical management applications. Laryngoscope 1996;106:97-101.

Burkart CM, Richter GT, Rutter MJ, Myer CM, 3rd. Update on endoscopic management of lingual thyroglossal duct cysts. Laryngoscope 2009;119:2055-60.

Chen EY, Inglis AF, Ou H, et al. Endoscopic electrocauterization of pyriform fossa sinus tracts as definitive treatment. Int J Pediatr Otorhinolaryngol 2009;73:1151-6.

Cotton RT. Management of subglottic stenosis. Otolaryngol Clin North Am 2000;33:111-30.

Derkay CS, Wiatrak B. Recurrent respiratory papillomatosis: a review. Laryngoscope 2008;118:1236-47.

DeSanto LW, Devine KD, Weiland LH. Cysts of the larynx--classification. Laryngoscope 1970;80:145-76.

Deutsch E, Kaufman M, Eilon A. Transnasal endoscopic management of choanal atresia. Int J Pediatr Otorhinolaryngol 1997;40:19-26.

Diamantopoulos, II, Jones NS. The investigation of nasal septal perforations and ulcers. J Laryngol Otol 2001;115:541-4.

Douglas R, Wormald PJ. Endoscopic surgery for juvenile nasopharyngeal angiofibroma: where are the limits? Curr Opin Otolaryngol Head Neck Surg 2006;14:1-5.

Franco LP, Camargos PA, Becker HM, Guimaraes RE. Nasal endoscopic evaluation of children and adolescents with cystic fibrosis. Braz J Otorhinolaryngol 2009;75:806-13.

Fu J, Xue X, Chen L, Fan G, Pan L, Mao J. Lingual thyroglossal duct cyst in newborns: previously misdiagnosed as laryngomalacia. Int J Pediatr Otorhinolaryngol 2008;72:327-32.

Garabedian EN, Pezzettigotta S, Leboulanger N, et al. Endoscopic surgical treatment of laryngotracheal clefts: indications and limitations. Arch Otolaryngol Head Neck Surg 2010;136:70-4.

Giacomini PG, Ferraro S, Di Girolamo S, Ottaviani F. Large Nasal Septal Perforation Repair by Closed Endoscopically Assisted Approach. Ann Plast Surg 2011;66(6):633-6.

Gluckman PG, Chu TW, van Hasselt CA. Neonatal vallecular cysts and failure to thrive. J Laryngol Otol 1992;106:448-9.

Gold SM, Gerber ME, Shott SR, Myer CM, 3rd. Blunt laryngotracheal trauma in children. Arch Otolaryngol Head Neck Surg 1997;123:83-7.

Gutierrez JP, Berkowitz RG, Robertson CF. Vallecular cysts in newborns and young infants. Pediatr Pulmonol 1999;27:282-5.

Harley EH. Pediatric congenital nasal masses. Ear Nose Throat J 1991;70:28-32.

Hartzell LD, Richter GT, Glade RS, Bower CM. Accuracy and safety of tracheoscopy for infants in a tertiary care clinic. Arch Otolaryngol Head Neck Surg 2010;136:66-9.

Hedlund G. Congenital frontonasal masses: developmental anatomy, malformations, and MR imaging. Pediatr Radiol 2006;36:647-62; quiz 726-7.

Hengerer AS, Brickman TM, Jeyakumar A. Choanal atresia: embryologic analysis and evolution of treatment, a 30-year experience. Laryngoscope 2008;118:862-6.

Holinger LD, Barnes DR, Smid LJ, Holinger PH. Laryngocele and saccular cysts. Ann Otol Rhinol Laryngol 1978;87:675-85.

Hughes GB, Sharpino G, Hunt W, Tucker HM. Management of the congenital midline nasal mass: a review. Head Neck Surg 1980;2:222-33.

Hulsmann AR, de Bont N, den Hollander JC, Borgstein JA. Hamartomas of the oro- and nasopharyngeal cavity in infancy: two cases and a short review. Eur J Pediatr 2009;168:999-1001.

Ishman S, Book DT, Conley SF, Kerschner JE. Plastic bronchitis: an unusual bronchoscopic challenge associated with congenital heart disease repair. Int J Pediatr Otorhinolaryngol 2003;67:543-8.

Jablon JH, Hoffman JF. Birth trauma causing nasal vestibular stenosis. Arch Otolaryngol Head Neck Surg 1997;123:1004-6.

Jatana KR, Oplatek A, Elmaraghy CA. Bilateral vestibular stenosis from nasal continuous positive airway pressure/cannula oxygen administration. Otolaryngol Head Neck Surg 2008;138:690-1.

Jatana KR, Oplatek A, Stein M, Phillips G, Kang DR, Elmaraghy CA. Effects of nasal continuous positive airway pressure and cannula use in the neonatal intensive care unit setting. Arch Otolaryngol Head Neck Surg 2010;136:287-91.

Karen M, Chang E, Keen MS. Auricular composite grafting to repair nasal vestibular stenosis. Otolaryngol Head Neck Surg 2000;122:529-32.

Kim B, Park SH, Min HS, Rhee JS, Wang KC. Nasal chondromesenchymal hamartoma of infancy clinically mimicking meningoencephalocele. Pediatr Neurosurg 2004;40:136-40.

Koeller KK, Alamo L, Adair CF, Smirniotopoulos JG. Congenital cystic masses of the neck: radiologic-pathologic correlation. Radiographics 1999;19:121-46; quiz 52-3.

Kuint J, Horowitz Z, Kugel C, Toper L, Birenbaum E, Linder N. Laryngeal obstruction caused by lingual thyroglossal duct cyst presenting at birth. Am J Perinatol 1997;14:353-6.

LaBagnara J, Jr. Cysts of the base of the tongue in infants: an unusual cause of neonatal airway obstruction. Otolaryngol Head Neck Surg 1989;101:108-11.

Lanier B, Kai G, Marple B, Wall GM. Pathophysiology and progression of nasal septal perforation. Ann Allergy Asthma Immunol 2007;99:473-9; quiz 80-1, 521.

Maturo S, Hartnick C. Initial experience using propranolol as the sole treatment for infantile airway hemangiomas. Int J Pediatr Otorhinolaryngol;74:323-5.

McGill TJ. Congenital anomalies of the larynx. London: Arnold Publisher; 2000.

McKenna M, Brodsky L. Extraesophageal acid reflux and recurrent respiratory papilloma in children. Int J Pediatr Otorhinolaryngol 2005;69:597-605.

McMurray JS, Holinger LD. Otolaryngic manifestations in children presenting with apparent life-threatening events. Otolaryngol Head Neck Surg 1997;116:575-9.

Moes CA, Izukawa T, Trusler GA. Innominate artery compression of the Trachea. Arch Otolaryngol 1975;101:733-8.

Pignatari SS, Liriano RY, Avelino MA, Testa JR, Fujita R, De Marco EK. Gastroesophageal reflux in patients with recurrent laryngeal papillomatosis. Braz J Otorhinolaryngol 2007;73:210-4.

Preciado D, Verghese S, Choi S. Aggressive bronchoscopic management of plastic bronchitis. Int J Pediatr Otorhinolaryngol;74:820-2.

Quesnel AM, Lee GS, Nuss RC, Volk MS, Jones DT, Rahbar R. Minimally invasive endoscopic management of subglottic stenosis in children: Success and failure. Int J Pediatr Otorhinolaryngol 2011;75:652–656.

Rahbar R, Nicollas R, Roger G, et al. The biology and management of subglottic hemangioma: past, present, future. Laryngoscope 2004;114:1880-91.

Rahbar R, Rouillon I, Roger G, et al. The presentation and management of laryngeal cleft: a 10-year experience. Arch Otolaryngol Head Neck Surg 2006;132:1335-41.

Ramadan H, Ortiz O. Congenital nasal pyriform aperture (bony inlet) stenosis. Otolaryngol Head Neck Surg 1995;113:286-9.

Ramsden JD, Campisi P, Forte V. Choanal atresia and choanal stenosis. Otolaryngol Clin North Am 2009;42:339-52, x.

Russell HM, Backer CL. Pediatric thoracic problems: patent ductus arteriosus, vascular rings, congenital tracheal stenosis, and pectus deformities. Surg Clin North Am;90:1091-113.

Rutter MJ, Cotton RT, Azizkhan RG, Manning PB. Slide tracheoplasty for the management of complete tracheal rings. J Pediatr Surg 2003;38:928-34.

Salvado AR, Wang MB. Treatment of complete nasal vestibule stenosis with vestibular stents and mitomycin C. Otolaryngol Head Neck Surg 2008;138:795-6.

Shah RK, Mora BN, Bacha E, et al. The presentation and management of vascular rings: an otolaryngology perspective. Int J Pediatr Otorhinolaryngol 2007;71:57-62.

Tahir N, Ramsden WH, Stringer MD. Tracheobronchial anatomy and the distribution of inhaled foreign bodies in children. Eur J Pediatr 2009;168:289-95.

Terano C, Miura M, Fukuzawa R, et al. Three Children with Plastic Bronchitis Associated with 2009 H1n1 Influenza Virus Infection. Pediatr Infect Dis J. 2011;30(1):80-2.

Thompson DM. Abnormal sensorimotor integrative function of the larynx in congenital laryngomalacia: a new theory of etiology. Laryngoscope 2007;117:1-33.

Triglia JM, Nicollas R. Nasal and sinus polyposis in children. Laryngoscope 1997;107:963-6.

Tzifa A, Robards M, Simpson JM. Plastic bronchitis; a serious complication of the Fontan operation. Int J Cardiol 2005;101:513-4.

Verret DJ, McClay J, Murray A, Biavati M, Brown O. Endoscopic cauterization of fourth branchial cleft sinus tracts. Arch Otolaryngol Head Neck Surg 2004;130:465-8.

Weber SA, Ferrari GF. Incidence and evolution of nasal polyps in children and adolescents with cystic fibrosis. Braz J Otorhinolaryngol 2008;74:16-20.

Zielnik-Jurkiewicz B, Olszewska-Sosinska O. The nasal septum deformities in children and adolescents from Warsaw, Poland. Int J Pediatr Otorhinolaryngol 2006;70:731-6.

Zur KB, Litman RS. Pediatric airway foreign body retrieval: surgical and anesthetic perspectives. Paediatr Anaesth 2009;19 Suppl 1:109-17.

Part 4

Concepts in Endoscopic Surgery

8

Endoscopic Monitoring of Postoperative Sinonasal Mucosa Wounds Healing

Ivana Pajić-Penavić

*Department of ENT, Head and Neck Surgery, General
Hospital "Dr Josip Benčević", Slavonski Brod
Croatia*

1. Introduction

Nasal epithelium lies on the basement membrane, situated on the lamina propria. Pseudostratified columnar (respiratory) epithelium is composed of four major types of cells: ciliated cells, nonciliate cells, goblet cells and basal cells, ensuring mucus production and transport, resorption of surface materials, and formation of new epithelial cells. Lamina propria consists of two layers of seromucous glands, i.e. superficial and deep layers. Just beneath the basement membrane, lymphocytes and plasma cells form a lymphoid layer.

Maintenance of normal ventilation/aeration of sinus spaces is necessary for normal functioning of paranasal sinuses. The sinus labyrinth spaces and ostia of various sinus areas can be visualized by use of endoscopic techniques, e.g., in functional endoscopic sinus surgery (FESS). Ventilation and normal sinus function can be maintained by this minimally invasive method. Endoscopic sinus surgery (ESS) is the superior surgical method of treatment for recurrent acute sinusitis, chronic sinusitis, obstructive nasal polyposis, extramucous fungal sinusitis, periorbital abscess, rhinoliquorrhea, antrochoanal polyp, foreign body extraction, mucocele, dacryocystorhinostomy, excision of various tumors of the sinuses, nose, anterior, middle and posterior cranial fossa, epistaxis control, optic nerve decompression, choanal atresia, and orbit decompression. . Functional endoscopic sinus surgery (FESS), a minimally invasive technique, remains the most widely accepted therapy for chronic rhinosinusitis (CRS) and nasal polyposis (NP) after failure of medical treatment. FESS aims to remove inflammatory mucosa and to restore both ventilation and drainage of the sinus cavities. However, healing quality significantly influences the functional outcome. The exact mechanism of mucosal healing after sinus operation remains unclear. Postoperative wound healing is a highly coordinated process that includes coagulation, i.e. clot formation, inflammatory stage, and tissue formation and remodeling. During the process of healing, the extracellular matrix of nasal mucosa may be directly influenced by the growth factor (GF), while the expression of GF receptors may influence the cell phenotype and its adhesion. Endoscopic observation of the nasal and sinus mucosa healing after FESS revealed four clinical stages: stage 1 characterized by the formation of abundant crusts, lasting for 1-10 days; stage 2 characterized by obstructive lymphedema, with pronounced swelling of residual mucosa, lasting for up to 30 days; stage 3 characterized by mesenchymal growth, when pale, edematous mucosa is transformed to red mucosa, lasting for up to 3 months; and stage 4 characterized by cicatrix formation, lasting for 3-6 months.

The duration of particular stages can be reduced or prolonged by postoperative treatment. Any derangement in the process of healing may result in the formation of hypertrophic scar or impaired tissue differentiation, thus reducing functioning capacity of the organ involved. Healing defects of the respiratory mucosa regularly lead to development of infection or obstruction scar formation, making revision surgery necessary. Iatrogenic complication after FESS appears in 5% to 30% of patients, and recurrence is reported in about 18% of patients (Tan BK. 2010). Proper treatment of postoperative cavity is a significant segment in the process of mucosal healing, and thus part of the FESS. Due knowledge of the healing stages can help recognize a mucosal healing impairment and introduce appropriate therapy depending on the stage of the healing process. The healing stages and planning of postoperative therapy after endoscopic sinus surgery are presented.

1.1 Structure of sinonasl cavity
The nasal cavity and sinuses are covered with respiratory epithelium which is composed of ciliated pseudostratified columnar epithelium (respiratory epithelium) composed of four major types of cells: ciliated cells, nonciliated cells, goblet cells and basal cells assuring mucus production and transports, absorbtion of surface materials and formation of new epithelial cells. The lamina propria consists of two layers of seromucous glands: the superficial layer is situated just underneath the epithelium and the deep layer is under the vascular layer. Just beneath the basement membrane, lymphocytes and plasma cells form a lymphoid layer. The basal cells are intermediate stem cells capable of differentiation into ciliated columnar or goblet cells. Occasional cuboidal and squamous cells are also found the epithelium. The columnar cells are 25μm long and 7μm wide, tapering to 2-4μm at the base. They are separated from each other by tight junctions. Each cell is always covered by 300-400 microvilli, and may or may not have cilia. Microvillies increase the surface area, thereby preventing drying. The number of cilia on each cell and size of the cilia varies between different species. The goblet cells produce mucus. The size and staining characteristics of the cell will depend on the phase of the secretory cycle of each individual cell. The number of cells varies throughout the nose and sinuses. On the septum, there is gradual increase in numbers passing from anterior to posterior and increase from superior to inferior. The seromucinous glands are found in the submucosa of the respiratory epithelium. They are relatively few in number and are more numerous in the mucosa near the choanae. The mucosa of the nasal cavity is much thicker than that of the sinuses. Mucosa tends to be thin and dry over bony excrescences and outcroppings that are characteristically notable over the nasal septum and in nasal valve area. Sinus mucosa is much thinner than that lining the rest of the nasal cavity. Epithelium tends to be lower; there are generally few goblet cells; and seromucinous glands are extremely scarce. The basement membrane is attenuated or not readily discernible and the lamina propria is often absent. The basic cells are columnar ciliated epithelial cells. They average 5μm long and 0.2μm thick and carry between 100 and 150 cilia on each luminal cell surface. Microvilli are much smaller, averaging around 1.5μm long and 0.08μm in diameter. Goblet cells are shorter except during the active phase of secretion. The maxillary sinus is lined with ciliated columnar respiratory epithelium containing goblet cells and glands. The mucous membrane is relatively thin, less vascular and more loosely adherent to the bony walls than in the nasal cavity. Density of goblet cells in the maxillary sinus is the highest of any in the paranasal sinuses, and similar to that on the inferior turbinate. There is no obvious increase in goblet cell density around the ostium. The seromucinous glands, though few in number compared with the goblet cells, are again

more numerous in the maxillary sinus compared with the other sinuses, and are more concentrated around the ostium. Ethmoid sinuses are also lined with ciliated columnar respiratory epithelium. The density of goblet cells is lower then in the maxillary sinus. Tubuloalveolar seromucinous glands are found trough out the mucosa and are actually more numerous in the ethmoid than in the other sinuses. In sphenoid sinuses the respiratory epithelium contains goblet cells and glands, as in the other sinuses. Goblet cells are of similar density as in the ethmoids, though the glands are last numerous in these sinuses and are therefore not found on all walls. The frontal sinus respiratory epithelium has the fewest number of goblet cells and very few glands. Mucus has a gel and sol layer with the narrow sol layer covering the cilia, facilitating their movement, and the gel layer on top to which foreign material will stick. Mucus blanket sweeps from the nares to the choanae and in the sinus cavities toward their ostia. The only exception to this is the frontal sinus in which the mucus blanket sweeps from the ostium, arcs over the roof of the sinus, and progresses along the floor to empty into the lateral aspect of the frontal sinus ostium. Vasculature of the nose is characterized by capacitance vessels. With these vascular specificities, nasal mucosa can regulate the airflow, adapt the nasal resistance, filter and condition the inspired air, and organize the first line of immune defense. Ethmoid bloc is the most complex of the sinuses. It often appears to be pivotal sinus in pathophysiology of sinus inflammatory disease (Donald PJ.1995).

1.2 Cytokines and GFs in nasal repair
The transforming growth factor-beta (TGF-β) is the most relevant growth factor in wound healing, affecting nearly all the phases of the process. Besides its immunosuppressive effects, TGF-β1 influences cell proliferation and myofibroblast differentiation. GFs are mediators produced by cells, tissue or blood products that activate target cells to proliferate by binding to their high-affinity surface membrane receptors. Transforming GF (TGF) β is released by major cell types participating in the repair process (epithelial cells, inflammatory cells, fibroblast, etc.) and nearly all cells express TGF-β receptors. More than 85% of TGF-β in adult wound fluid is of the type 1 isoform. TGF-β had important activities such as an adverse effect in vitro on reepithelization, immunosuppression, or stimulation of ECM deposition. PDGF isoforms have potent mitogenic and chemotactic activities on dermal fibroblasts, endothelial cells, smooth muscle cells, neutrophils, and macrophages and stimulates collagen synthesis and collagenase acitivity. PDGF isoforms have potent mitogenic and cemotactic activities on fibroblasts, endothelial cells, smooth muscle cells.

Epidermal GF (EGF) family, including aphiregulin and TGF-α has been shown to induce epithelial development and differentiation, to promote angiogenesis, and, in vivo, to accelerate wound healing. Cells associated with wound healing such as inflammatory cells (macrophages and T lymphocytes), vascular endothelial cells, and fibroblasts can produce fibroblast GF (FGF), which are mitogens for a wide variety cell types. Insulin-like GF (IGF) I and II have an amino acid sequence homologous to proinsulin and are secreted by a wide range of adult tissues. IGF-I (known as Somatomedin-C) stimulates, in vitro mitosis of fibroblasts, osteocytes and chondrocytes. Because its combination with other growth hormones is more effective than either peptide alone, it frequently acts in synergy with PDGF to enhance epidermal regeneration. GFs enhance the deposition of extracellular matrix (ECM). Extracellular matrix provides nutrients support, and adhesion for the inflammatory on structural cells participating in repair (Watelet JB. 2002).

1.3 Neutrophils in wound healing

Neutrophils play an important role in tissue remodeling occurring after tissue damage. The particular inverse relationship between eosinophils and fibrosis found at baseline persists during the healing process. On the other hand, macrophages and eosinophil cells are highly associated not only with the tissue remodeling characteristic of chronic sinus disease but also with the neutrophilic inflammation occurring during wound repair. Macrophages and eosinophil cells were highly associated not only with the tissue remodeling characteristic of chronic sinus diseases but also with the neutrophilic inflammation occurring during wound repair. The selective recruitment of eosinophils into sinonasal inflamed tissue involves priming, activation, and recruitment mediated by chemoattractants, cell adhesion molecules, and cytokines. Activated eosinphils contribute to the production of cytokines and inflammatory molecules, which damage nasal mucosa, leading to edema and inflammation. The differentiation of mast cells occurs by the effects of released cytokines from inflammatory cells. Histamine, prostaglandine E2, and leukotriens are released from degranulate mast cells. Sensory nerve stimulation by these mediators attracts eosinophils to the inflammatory areas. Substance P released by mast cells causes increased vasodilatation, increased vascular permeability, mucous secretion, and eosinophil chemotaxis; increase mast cells degranulation; and enhances the response to allergens in atopics patients (Watelet JB. 2006).

1.3.1 Neutrophil-derived Metalloproteinase-9

Metalloproteinase-9 (MM-9) expression in ECM was also significantly correlated with healing quality. MM-9 is actively expressed by eosinophils, monocytes-macrophages, epithelial-derived cells and is stored by neutrophils. It degrades collagen fibres, basement membrane, fibronectin and elastin. MM-9 activity is controlled at different levels: transcription of the gene under control of cytokines or cellular interaction, activation of the proenzyme by serin proteases or other MMPs, and finally, activity regulation by natural tissue inhibitors (TIMPs). The amounts of MMP-9 in nasal fluid are linked to ECM expression of MMP-9. The MMP-9 deposition inside ECM correlates with inflammatory cells. The number of neutrophils and lesser extent, macrophages could predict MMP-9 release in nasal fluid. There is close relationship between MMP-9 and neutrophils and they establish a direct link between the severity of the inflammatory reaction and the consequent tissue damage. MMP-9 is considered as effector but also as a regulator of leukocyte function. It is stored in granules of mature neutrophils and has been shown to be a specific marker of neutrophils and has been shown to be a specific marker of neutrophils maturation. Transcription of the gelatinase-B gene is stimulated in leukocytes by cytokines, viral or bacterial products, or cellular interactions. In response to lipopolysaccharide, the neutrophil is responsible for the rapid secretion of MMP-9 as a result of release of preformed enzymes stored in granules. The level of MMPs parallels the severity of clinical condition. Release of gelatinase-B by degranulation of neutrophils occurs within the first hour when these cells are stimulated by chemotactic factors. During wound healing, the association beween neutrophils and macrophages observed in tissue suggests that the amounts of MMP-9 requested are high and that a conjunction of rapid release and continuous production is needed. MMP-9 has been shown to clip many cytokines or chemokines such as interleukin (IL) -1β or IL-8. On the other hand, the binding of MMP-9 to the plasma membrane of neutrophils enables it to be inhibited by TIMPs and thereby may alter the pericellular proteolytic balance in favor of ECM degradation. The MMP-9 production by neutrophils participates actively in airway remodeling (Watelet JB. 2005)

2. General principles of wound healing

Wound healing of the mucosa lining consists a few phases such as: inflammation, cell proliferation, matrix deposition and remodeling (Watelet JB.2002).

2.1 Coagulation

Injury to the nasal epithelium causes hemorrhage with exposure of platelets to the connective tissue, which activates the platelets and results in an almost immediate release of numerous vasoactive substances (serotonin, bradykinin and histamine). The subsequent transient (5-10 minutes) vasoconstriction helps to control bleading and is followed by the formation of a primary hemostatic plug with aggregation of platelets in the mucosal effect. Platelets are critical elements during this early response, not only because of their concurrent release of numerous cytokines. Damaged nasal cells release PDGF, TGF-α and TGF- β and mast cells represent another source of biologically active substance or GFs that regulate the early repair sequences. Fibrin, in conjunction with fibronectin, acts as a provisional matrix for the influx of monocytes and fibroblasts. Fibrin also stimulates the α-granules within the aggregated platelets to release PDGF, EGF, IGF-I, TGF-β and FGF.

2.2 Inflamation

In the nasal lamina propria, an intense inflammatory reaction starts simultaneously with the coagulation phase. This inflammation is marked by an infiltration of leukocytes, which migrate through vessel walls by a process known as diapedesis. Polymorphonuclear neutrophils predominate during the first 24-48 hours and stimulate release of elastase and collagenase molecules, which facilitate cell penetration into the ECM. Three to five days after injury, the neutrophilic population in the wound is replaced by monocyte predominance. Unlike neutrophils, the influx of macrophages is essential for the continuation of nasal wound repair. Macrophages contribute to cellular debridement and secret a number of GFs: TGF-β, basic FGF (b FGF), EGF, TGF-α and PDGF. They amplify and sustain the wound healing process. Lymphocytes and their products, TGF-β, interleukin, tumor necrosis factor and interferons also interact with the macrophages during the inflammatory process, linking the immune response to wound healing. In a typically clean surgical wound, this inflammatory reaction subsides over a period of several days.

2.3 Tissue formation

New stroma or granulation tissue consisting of fibroblasts, macrophages and neovasculature can be observed 4 days after injury within a loose connective tissue matrix of collagen, hyaluronic acid and fibronectin. Macrophages of the nasal lamina propria provide a continuing source of cytokines necessary to stimulate proliferation of fibroblast and angiogenesis.

2.3.1 Fibroplasia

This term reflects fibroblast cell migration or proliferation and ECM deposition. Through a variety of cytokines from platelets and macrophages or through an autocrine regulation, fibroblasts are attracted to the nasal wound. Structural molecules of the early ECM also contribute to tissue formation by providing a network for cell mobility and guidance (fibronectin, collagen and hyaluronic acid) and by acting as a cytokine reservoir. Once the nasal fibroblasts have migrated into the wound, they gradually switch their major function to protein synthesis and GF release. The composition and structure of granulation tissue depends both on the time course since tissue injury and on the distance from the wound margin.

2.3.2 Angiogenesis
Nasal endothelial cells start to proliferate through fragmented basement membranes. They migrate into the perivascular space, and other endothelial cells follow. Angiogenic GFs: FGF, TGF-β, EGF, TGF -α and PDGF, released from injured nasal cells, platelets and ECM, induced vascularization, resulting in delivering oxygen to the wound bed. Endothelial cell migration depends on continuous collagen secretion and is accompanied by proteoglycan synthesis.

2.3.3 Reepithelization
Migration of new respiratory cells from the undamaged areas starts within a few hours, with an estimated velocity of 4μm/hour in the sinuses. The nasal epithelial cells at the wound edge lose their apical-basal polarity and develop cytoplasmic extensions into the wound. Four different processes are operative during regeneration: migration from adjacent epithelium, multiplication of undifferentiated cells, reorientation and differentiation. Undifferentiated respiratory basal cells from adjacent non-traumatized areas seem to serve as the main source of new cells. Different hypotheses are proposed to explain the initiation of reepithelialization: absence of neighbor cells at the wound margin, local release of GFs (TGF-α and EGF) or increase of GF receptors.

2.4 Tissue remodeling
Nasal ECM remodeling, cell maturation and cell apoptosis overlapping with tissue formation and wound remodeling may continue up to 6 month after surgery. Most cells produce proteinases able to degrade the ECM. These enzymes can be subdivided into three groups: the serine proteinase, the matrix metalloproteinases ad the cysteine proteinase (cathepsins). The matrix metalloproteinases need an active Zn+ site for their catalytic mechanism and they can be categorized in function of their degradation abilities in the ECM: interstitial collagenases 1-3, stromelysins 1-3, gelatinases A and B, matrilysin, macrophage metalloelastase and transmembrane metalloproteinase. Their proteolytic activity is controlled by tissue-erived metalloproteinase inhibitors 1-3.

In the remodeling or maturation phase, the inflammators response and angiogenesis diminish, whereas the intense fibroblast proliferation starts to attenuate. The composition of ECM changes as the wound matures. Initially, The ECM is composed mainly of hyaluronic acid, fibronectin and collagen types I, III and V. During remodeling, the ratio of collagen type I to III changes until type I is the dominant form; elastin fibers or proteglycans are actively produced within the matrix. This dynamic balance between collagen synthesis and lysis is responsible for the maturation of the wound. This phase increases wound tensile strength and resilience to deformation.

3. Endoscopic observations of wound healing

Endoscopic observation of normal wound healing revealed four different phases (Hosemann W. 1991, Xu G.2008):

3.1 I Phase of blood crusting (day 1-10)

During the first stage / peak the operative cavity is clean or dry, which is called "*stage of clean cavity*". In the 3-5 days after the filled nasal material was taken away, oozed blood clotted and formed a dry and hard black crust. During the first 10 days the endoscopic picture was dominated by blood crusts. After 12th days the whole wound was covered by blood crusts. There was no change of the residual mucosa underneath these crusts within the first 2-3 days. Due to shortage of mucosa clearance, viscous secretion was gathered in the bottom of the sinus, and mucosa gap and fibrous pseudomembrane was observed on the surface of mucosa with responsive edema. The edematous swelling became more marked after detachment of the crusts in the second phase. On days 7-10, the edema was relieved and secretion was reduced, and clots and crusts decreased or disappeared after cleaning. After 10 days, the operative cavity became clean.

3.2 II Phase of obstructive lymphedema (up t 30 days)

During this period, the residual mucosa showed edematous swelling. This is secondary peak which occurs in the third to tenth weeks. Edema reoccurred in the operative cavity mainly due to lymphatic obstruction. Vesicles, mini-polyps and granulation tissue began to grow in the mucosa gap, which is called "*reaction to mucosa removal*". Hyperplasia and adhesion of connective tissue were also observed in this stage. In the meantime, regeneration and epithelialization were also happening, competing against mucosa diseases. After the vesicles, granulation tissue, mini-polyps and fibrous adhesion had been cleaned and mucosa regeneration and epithelialization expanded little by little, the scope of disease got smaller and smaller, and complete epithelialization was attained in the end. This secondary edema regresses spontaneously. If this phase is not handled carefully, the diseases would expande gradually and hamper epithelialization, resulting in deferred inflammation, leading to adhesion, constriction and blockage of the operative cavity and sinus ostium. In view of stage characterized by coexistence and rivalry of mucosa regeneration and disease, it is called "*stage of mucosal transitional competition*". The generation of vesicles or polyps during this stage was simply regarded as "recurrence of disease" instead of an inevitable mucosal transitional process. When the local reaction to mucosal removal was under control, mucosa restored well.

3.3 III Phase of mesenchymal growth (up to 3 months)

After the 30th day, mucosal reorganization took place preferably below the regenerated epithelial covering. This is the third stage/ peak. After 10 weeks, implying finished epithelialization of the operative cavity, which was called "stage of complete epithelialization". Though epithelialization started in the first 2 weeks and extended to the second stage, only a small number of cases finished epithelialization within 5 weeks, the majority was after 10 weeks and had a benign outcome. The color of the mucosa changed from a yellowish-pale edema to a more reddish color.

Infection with additional destruction of the mucosa or excessive granulation allergic factors, hyperplasia of connective tissue and lack of control of regenerated polyps could slow down this epithelialization.

3.4 IV Phase of scarification (after 3 months)

At this time reorganization of tissue in the operated area had nearly finished. Subepithelial changes are noted after 6 months.

During these four phases in operative field can be seen:

1. *Clean cavity*: no oozing, fibrous pseudomembrane nearly disappeared, secretion decreased, clots and brown-yellow crusts diminished or disappeared
2. *Mucosal edema*: the whole inflammatory cavity and mucosa swelled, with smooth surface and indistinct boundary
3. *Edematous vesicle*: single or multiple or patches of polyp-like edematous vesicle appeared, with a grey, smooth and thin wall.
4. *Polyp*: it exists singly and locally
5. *Granulation tissue*: local or scattered hyperplasia occurred, with unsmooth papillary-like surface, fragile and easy to bleed
6. *Polyp-like mucosal edema*: extensive polyp-like changes and severe mucosal edema with plenty of purulent secretion were found
7. *Cicatricial tissue hyperplasia*: extensive connective tissue was yielded, mostly connected to patches, which was thick, tough and easy bleeding
8. *Adhesion*: fibrous membranous or cicatricial bridges resulted, mostly lying between the anterior verge of the middle turbinate and the lateral wall of the nasal cavity
9. *Empyema*: mostly was a viscous purulent secretion difficult to exudate
10. *Narrow or blocked sinus ostium*: fibrous cicatricial bridges occurred around the sinus ostium or connective tissue hyperplasia appeared
11. *Constriction and blockage of sinus cavity*: caused by adhesion of the laterally moved middle turbinate or connective tissue hyperplasia of the sinus wall
12. *Epithellization*: thin and smooth mucosa was found, which was closely linked with the preserved sinus bone wall and anatomical processes, and well-opened sinus ostia were clearly observed.

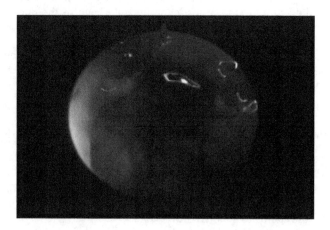

Fig. 1. Clean cavity (blood clot)

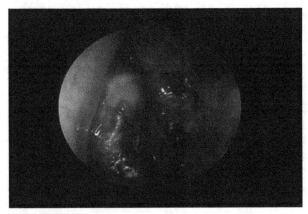

Fig. 2. Clean cavity (hard black crusts)

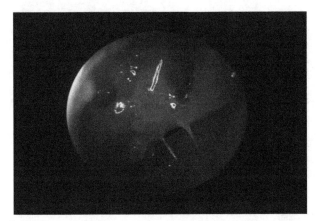

Fig. 3. Mucosal edema

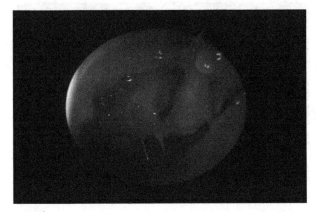

Fig. 4. Edematous vesicle

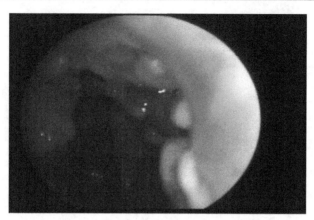

Fig. 5. Polyp formation

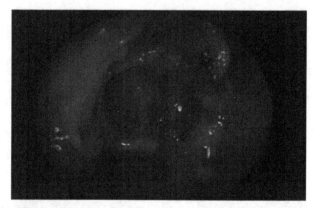

Fig. 6. Granulation tissue

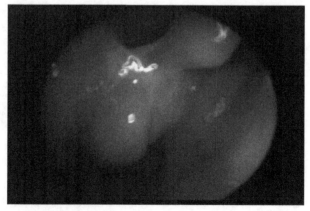

Fig. 7. Polyp like mucosal edema

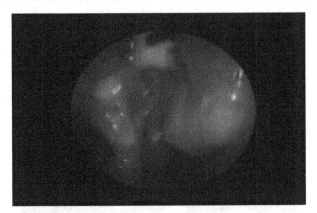

Fig. 8. Cicatrical tissue

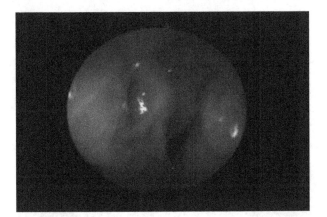

Fig. 9. Adhesion

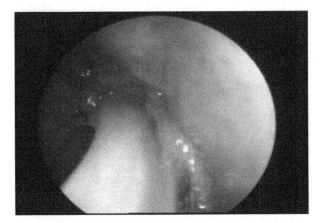

Fig. 10. Empyema

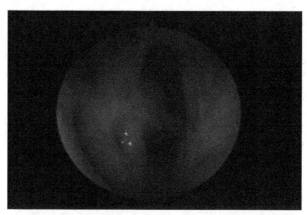

Fig. 11. Narrow or blocked sinus cavity

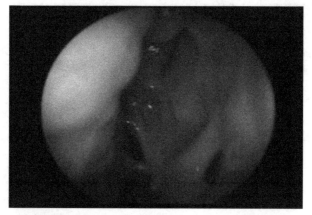

Fig. 12. Constriction and blockage of sinus cavity

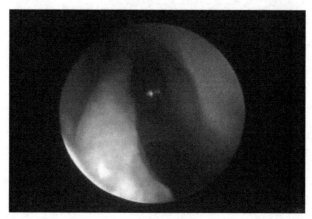

Fig. 13. Epithelization

Clinical observations of wound healing in human beings have shown predisposed areas of reduced healing, suggesting that local microanatomical factors may play a decisive role in the reparation process. The closure of a defined wound of the respiratory mucous membrane is independent of the direction of blood, lymph or mucociliary flow. The management of the operative cavity especially in the first and second stages was essential to the whole curative effect, making up an important part of ESS.

Functional postoperative results are directly dependent on the healing quality of the nasal or sinusal mucosa and it can end differently. If the healing is dominant it can end with completed epithelial metaplasia, but if there is dominance of regenerative phase, epithelial metaplasia will be incomplete with adhesion, partial or total obstruction of the ostium and sinus cavity. Despite advances in instrumentation and surgical technique, postoperative synechia formation continues to occur in between 1-27% of patients. When sinechia occur in the middle meatus, the maxillary, ethmoid and frontal sinuses may become obstructed resulting in recurrent problems. The reported complications following ESS can be classified broadly into immediate postoperative complications such as bleeding and crusting; short-term complications such as infection, synechiae formation, and turbinate lateralization; and long-term complications such as ostial stenosis, refractory disease, and disease recurrence.

Mucosal sparing techniques, middle turbinate resection or medialization and frequent postoperative debridement have been used to varying degrees and with varying success to prevent postoperative synechia.

4. Principles of management in different stages after operation

Different author suggests different time of postoperative observation and care after extensive paranasal surgery. It is from 1 to 12 month. The crucial care of postoperative sinonasal mucosa is topical care and it should be:

Nasal packing, whether absorbable or nonabsorbable, has little effect on postoperative bleeding but more importantly, plays a more important role in postoperative healing. Considering the average duration of postoperative bleeding and the infection risk because of the " foreign body" there is no reason to leave a packing for more than 3 days. Blood surrounding the packing may (re)organize and the fibrin deposits around the packing could lead to scar tissue and adhesions. Packing moreover may obstruct evacuation of blood and secretions from the paranasal sinuses (Jorissen M. 2004.). Gelatin antibiotic and glucocorticosteroid can accelerate mucosa regeneration.

Rinse with enzymes contributes to the dissolution of fibrous pseudo membrane, clots and crusts, thus promoting the cleaning and healing of the sinus mucosa. Irrigation with saline solution is conductive to improve local nasal blood circulation and ciliary clearance. Using small volume (up to 1ml) only dampens the nasal mucosa, and the paranasal sinuses can not be reached. Only with large volume (300ml for a nose can) can the paranasal sinuses be reached, rinsed and washed. In addition to the pure mechanical rinsing, the saline will mix with secretions and decrease viscosity, propagating evacuation by mucociliary transport. High volume-low pressure rinsing of the nose and paranasal sinuses is the preferred technique for cleaning the surgical cavity and improving wound healing (Jorissen 2004). Welch recently published a study of the irrigation bottles used by patients after ESS and found that bacteria could be cultured from the irrigation bottles in 29% of studied patients including *Pseudomonas aerugionosa, Acinetobacter baumanni,* and *Klebsiella pneumoniae* although fortunately no clinically significant postoperative infections were noted. Frequent changing and sterilization of nasal irrigation bottles is advocated (Welch2009). Nasal irrigation with sulfurous-arsenical-ferruginous solution locally reduce the eosinophil number and may limit eosinophil-mediated production of cytokines and inflammatory molecules, which damage nasal mucosa, leading to edema and sinonasl inflammation. As eosinophils play an important role in allergic response through the release of mediators as eosinophilic cationic protein, major basic protein, and leukotrien C4, which causes extracellular matrix deposition, epithelial denudation, and basement membrane disruption. Sulfurous-arsenical ferruginous solution nasal irrigation significantly reducing the local eosinophil count should be suggested for allergic patients (Staffieri A. 2008). Local steroid spray has potent regional anti-allergy anti-inflammatory and anti-edema effects, which can control the generation of vesicles and mini polyps. The incidence of morphological changes in the nasal mucosa of patients with perennial rhinitis following treatment for 1 year with MFNS (mometasone furoate nasal spray) 100-200µg b.i.d. has demonstrated that this agent did not lead to any significant adverse tissue changes including increase in epithelial thickness or tissue atrophy, although the numbers of inflammatory cells in the epithelium and lamina propria were significantly decreased, compared to baseline (Minshall E. 1998). Subjects with an initial diagnosis of nasal polyps (CRSwNP) were more likely to experience MFNS-mediated improvements in wound healing than subjects with an initial diagnosis of chronic rhinosinusitis without polyposis (CRSsNP). At a subcellular level, corticosteroids have an antiinflammatory effect by activating glucocorticoid receptors,which interact with inflammatory transcription factors resulting in suppression of proinflammatorymolecules. At a cellular level, corticosteroids reduce the quantity of inflammatory cells (eosinophils, T lymphocytes,mast cells, and dendritic cells), the degree of inflammatory suppression correlates with the tissue concentration of steroid (Jorissen M. 2009). Oral steroids used preoperatively in patients undergoing endoscopic sinus surgery for nasal polyposis have been shown to reduce vascularity and improve surgical nasal field conditions resulting in shorter operating time. Postoperative administration of intranasal corticosteroids has also been demonstrated to reduce nasal polyp recurrence after endoscopic sinus surgery. The effect of oral steroids was investigated in the UZ Leuven in prospective, randomized comparative study: 1 tablet of betamethasone 0,25mg during 20 days versus a reducing regimen (4co/d d1-d5, 3co/d d5-d10, 2co/d d11-d15 and finally 1 co/d d16-d20). For all groups of patients beneficial effects of a higher dose of steroids during the first 3 weeks after ESS were found and the systemic and local side effects of the higher dose oral regimen were minor (Jorissen 2004). Gelomyrtol forte capsules are conductive to loosen viscous mucus secretion, dissolve fibrous adhesion and increase mucociliary clearance. Inhibitor of proton pump once / at night or twice a day is recommended to reduce gastric fluid acidity. Gastroesophageal reflux may play a significant role in wound healing. This is illness that includes the most of population. In GERB the lower esophageal sphincter doesn't work well, but in LPR (laryngopharyngeal reflux) the problem is in upper esophageal sphincter. Laryngopharyngeal reflux is defined as the retrograde movement of gastric contents into the larynx, pharynx, and upper aerodigestive tract. Mucosa of the respiratory tract is more sensitive on acid and pepsin instead of esophageal mucosa. Acids can locally harm the mucosa and increase mucosal reaction that leads to prolonged inflammation with granulation. Night reflux phases are much longer than day phases and they can lead to mucosal damages. The nasal symptoms aggravate during nights and in the mornings which can be connected with LPR. So, LPR can aggravate healing of sinonasal mucosa (Kleemann 2005).

Crusting or cloting may trap mucus, resulting in reinfection of the sinuses, and the old blood itself may serve as a culture medium for bacteria. The crusts may act as bridges in which scar formation may occur, leading to an obstructed postoperative cavity and synechia formation in the middle meatus. Retained bone fragments that are denuded of mucosa may act as base for reinfection. Removing the crust, suctioning the retained secretion, and preventing lateral synechia formation and the obstruction of ostia and air cells are essential for healing and successful surgical outcome. Blood crusts cover the mucosal wound in the first 2 to 3 weeks and mucosal edema continues about 4 to 6 weeks after the operation. Although frequent postoperative debridement may remove the loose crusts and small devitalized bone fragments. Hard or fixed crusts cannot be cleaned because of bleeding from the underlying mucosal surface, discomfort and pain, and reformation of blood crusts. Loose, removable crusts were observed 2 weeks after the operation, indicating that mucosal re-epithelization requires at least 2 weeks. Mucosal edema was increased and sustained for 4 to 6 weeks. Mechanical wound care and the removal of blood crusts was avoided for at least 10 days. Gentle suction cleaning for several mounts. Violent tearing and too much cutting, which may cause injury to the epithelium, should be avoided. Sharp curette, electric cutter (debrider) and laser are recommended to lean the regenerated lesions. During the process of epithelization, the sinus was managed once at week, and any invalid surgery should be avoided unless the above-mentioned diseases occur because newly formed epithelium is loosely connected to bone, which is easy to tear away (Lee JY. 2008). The postoperative cleaning should continue until the operative site is mucosally covered. Presence of cultured bacteria from post-ESS patient cavities remains unclear. Several investigators have described the presence of biofilms in post-ESS cavities, and a retrospective pathologic study by Psaltis found that bacterial biofilms were found in 20 (50%) of the 40 CRS patients. Patients with biofilms also had significantly worse preoperative radiological scores and, postoperatively, had statistically worse postoperative symptoms and mucosal outcomes (Psaltis AJ. 2008). The use of an antibiotic (amoxicillin/clavulanate) in the postoperative period is able to improve the outcome in the early blood crust healing phase: nasal obstruction and drainage are reduced and the endoscopic score objectively showed a faster recovery (Albu S. 2010). Patients recover in 9 to 10 days after ESS when provided with appropriate pain management. Postoperative pain after ESS can be controlled effectively with acetaminophen 665mg modified-release tablets three times a day during the first five postoperative days (Kempainen TP. 2007). Postoperative treatment after endoscopic surgery of frontal sinus or frontal recess is a little bite different of others sinuses. No nasal packing needs to be used. The frontal sinus cannulae are left in place for up to 5 days if there has been inadvertent trauma to the frontal ostium mucosa, if the natural frontal sinus ostium is very narrow (<3mm), if there was evidence of osteitis with new bone formation in the frontal recess or ostium, and if there was extensive polyposis resulting in significant traumatized mucosa after the polyp removal. Frontal sinus saline douches are started through the frontal cannulae within 2 hours of completion of the operation. This will wash any blood clot out of the frontal ostium. The frontal cannulae are flushed with 5mL normal saline every 2 hours starting immediately after surgery. If prednisolone drops are to be used 0, 5 to 1mL is instilled with a syringe into the frontal sinus after every second douche. The aim of the prednisolone is to dampen the inflammatory response of the mucosa. Immediately prior to removal of the frontal sinus cannulae, 5mL of steroid and antibiotic cream (not ointment) is injected through each cannulae. This coats the newly created frontal sinus ostium and tends to decrease the amount of adherent crusts (Wormald PJ2008). Every operation, no matter how minor, is accompanied by swelling of the surrounding tissues. The amount of swelling varies from person to person, but it always seems more dramatic when involving the face. We suggest that you keep your head elevated as much as possible. The swelling itself is normal and is not an indication that something is wrong with the healing phase of your operation. Swelling after sinus surgery is not usually seen on the face itself; rather, it manifests itself as a stuffy or blocked nasal passage. Any swelling of the face will be limited to the area around the eyes and will last for only a few days. Symptoms of pain and pressure will be relieved in the very early postoperative period while thick postnasal drainage will continue until the mucosa within the sinuses has returned to normal. This may take weeks to months depending on the severity of the disease and the rapidity of healing. The patients should be warned of this preoperatively.

Proposed therapy

1. The packing, tamponades, should be removed from first till fifth day (as soon as possible)
2. Irrigation with saline solution 3 times a day for 3 weeks, high volume (>100ml), low pressure rinsing
3. Irrigation with sulfurous-arsenical-ferruginous solution for 3 weeks (for patients who has allergy)
4. The frontal cannulae are flushed with 5mL normal saline every 2 hours starting immediately after surgery and Prednisolon drops 0, 5 to 1mL instilled with syringe into the frontal sinus after every second douche (for frontal Sinus surgery)
1. Rinse with enzymes can promote cleaning and healing of sinus mucosa
2. Bloody sediment and the crusts in the nasal cavity should drained with sucker after 10th day
3. Endoscopic treatment once a week in weeks 2-6
4. Topical drugs: glucocorticosteroids nasal spray apply once or twice- daily for 6 months (for patients who has allergy)
5. Topical drugs: glucocorticosteroids can stop once healing has occur (for patients who has no other problems than chronic infection)
6. Oral glucocorticosteroids: Prednison 1mg/kg 5 days before surgery and higher dose of steroids during the first 3 weeks (for patients with nasal polyposis)
7. Mucus eliminator such as Gelomyrtol forte capsules are recommended for 10 weeks
8. Proton pump inhibitors once / at night or twice a day is recommended to reduce gastric fluid acidity for 3 months (for patients who has LPR)
9. Pain killer, Acetaminophen 665mg modified-release tablets three times a day for first 5 days
10. Antibiotics (Amoxicillin/Clavulanate) for 2 weeks

Some tips to shorten the duration of the swelling and improve the ability to breathe through your nose include:

1. Stay vertical. Sit, stand and walk around as much as is comfortable beginning on your second postoperative day. Of course, you should rest when you become tired but keep your upper body as upright as possible.
2. Gentle blowing of the nose is allowed without closing the nasal vestibule.
3. Avoid bending over or lifting heavy things for one week. In addition to aggravating swelling, bending and lifting may elevate blood pressure and start bleeding.
4. Sleep with the head of the bed elevated 45 degrees for 7 – 10 days following your surgery. To accomplish this, place two or three pillows under the head of the mattress and one or two on top of the mattress. It is helpful if you sleep on your back for 30 nights.

5. Avoid straining during elimination. If you need a laxative. Proper diet, plenty of water and walking are strongly recommended to avoid constipation.
6. Avoid sunning of your face for one month. Always use a sunscreen with SPF15 or above.
7. Avoid exercise for one week following surgery.

5. References

Albu S, Lucaciu R. Prophylactic antibiotics in endoscopic sinus surgery: a short follow up study. *Am J. Rhinol Allergy*.2010; 24:306-9.

Donald PJ, Gluckman JL, Rice DH (1995) The Sinuses. *Raven Press New York, ISBN 0-7817-0041-8.*

Hosemann W, Wigand ME, Göde U, Länger F, Dunker I (June1990) Normal wound healing of the paranasal sinuses: clinical and experimental investigations. *Eur Arch Otorhinolaryngol*, 1991; 248:390-394.

Jorissen M (2004) Postoperative care following endoscopic sinus surgery.*Rhinology*, 2004;42:114-120.

Jorissen M, Bschert C (December 2008) Efects of corticosteroids on wound healing after endoscopic sinus sugery.*Rhinology*, 2009;47: 280-286. DOI:10.4193/Rhin08.227.

Kemppainen TP, Toumilehto H, Kokki H, Seppä J, Nuutinen J. Pain treatment and recovery after endoscopic sinus surgery. *Laryngoscope*, 2007; 117:1434-8.

Kleeman D, Nofz S, Plank I, Schlottmann A (November 2004) Prolongierte Heilungsverläufe nach endonasalen Nasen-nebenhöhlenoperationen. *HNO*, 2005; 53:333-36.DOI 10.1007/s00106-004-1108y.

Lee JY, Byun JY. Relationship between the frequency of postoperative debridement and patient discomfort, healing period, surgical outcomes, and compliance after endoscopic sinus surgery.*Larynoscope*, 2008;118:1868-72. DOI: 10.1097/MLGOb013e31817f93d3.

Minshall E, Ghaffar O, Cameron L (1998) Assesment by nasal biopsy of long –term use of mometasone furoate aqueous nasal spray in the treatment of perennial rhinitis. *Otolaryngol Head Neck Surg*, 118: 648-654.

Psaltis AJ, Weitzel EK, Ha KR (2008) The effect of bacterial biofilms on postsinus surgical outcomes. *Am J Rhinol* 2008; 22:1-6.

Xu G, Jiang H, Li H, Shi J, Chen H (April 2008) Stages of nasal mucosal transitional course after functional endoscopic sinus surgery and their clinical indications *ORL*,2008;70:118-123. DOI: 10.1159/0014535.

Staffieri A, Marino F Staffieri C, Giacomelli L, D´Alessandro D, Ferraro SM, Fedrazzoni U, Marioni G (2008) The effects of sulphurous-arsenical ferruginous thermal water nasal irrigation in wound healing after functional endoscopic sinus surgery for chronic rhinosinusitis: a prospective randomized study. *American Journal of Otolaryngology-Head and Neck Medicine Surgery*, 2008; 29:223-229.

Tan BK, Chandra RK (2010) Postoperative prevention and treatment of complications after sinus suregry. *Otolaryngol Clin N Am*.2010; 43: 769-779. DOI: 10.1016/j.otc.2010.04.004.

Watelet JB, Gevaert P, Bachart C (Avgust 2001) Secretion of TGF-ß1, TGF-ß2, EGF and PDGF into nasal fluid after sinus surgery. *Eur Arch Otorhinolaryngol*, 2002; 259:234-238. DOI: 10.1007/s00405-002-0448-z.

Watelet JB, Bachert C, Gevaert P, Van Cauwenberge P (2002) Wound Healing of the nasal and paranasal mucosa: A review. *American Journal of Rhinology*, 2002; 16: 77-84.

Watelet JB, Demeter P, Claeys C, Van Cauwenberge P, Cuvelier C, Bachert C (2005) Neutrophil-derived Metalloprotenase-9 predicts healing quality after sinus surgery. *The laryngoscope*, 2005; 115:56-61. DOI: 10.1097/01.mlg.0000150674.30237.3f.

Watelet JB, Demetter P, Claeys C, Van Cauwenberge P, Cuvelier C, Bachert C (April 2005) Wound healing after paranasal sinus surgery: neutrophilic inflammation influences the outcome. *Histopatology*, 2006; 48: 174-181.D=I: 10.1111(j.1365-2559.2005.02310.x

Welch KC, Cohen MB, Doghramji LL (2009). Clinical correlation between irrigation bottle contamination and clinical outcomes in postfunctional endoscopic sinus surgery patients. *Am J Rhinol Allergy.*2009; 23:401-4.

Wormald PJ (2008). Endoscopic sinus surgery anatomy,three-dimensional reconstruction and surgical technique. Second edition. *Thieme New York. Stuttgart,* The Americas ISBN:978-1-58890-603-8, Rest of World ISBN: 978-3-13-139422-4.

9

Laparoscopic Surgery: An Almost Scarless Approach

Peng Soon Koh and Kin Fah Chin
Department of Surgery, Faculty of Medicine,
University of Malaya, Kuala Lumpur
Malaysia

1. Introduction

Minimally invasive surgery is gaining popularity worldwide as it contributes to less post-operative pain, shorter hospital stay and reduced morbidity. Since laparoscopic cholecystectomy was first performed in the 80's, a wide array of different types of laparoscopic surgery was performed and this has been extended to colorectal resection, where the first reported case of laparoscopic colorectal resection was made in 1991. Conventionally, a mini laparotomy is required to extract the specimen following laparoscopic colorectal resection, which may increase post-operative pain, wound infection, a bigger scar and other pain related morbidities. Thus, the use of natural orifice specimen extraction (NOSE) for the extraction of colorectal specimen is slowly gaining worldwide acceptance and evolving.

Single Incision laparoscopic Surgery or Single Port Access Surgery is also gaining popularity as an alternative approach to NOSE and Natural Orifice Transluminal Endoscopic Surgery (NOTES) in order to provide an almost scarless surgery. Often at times, such procedures are complementary to one another.

However, there is a significant cost implication due to the expensive disposable port and hand instruments but the main aim of having such procedures is the retrieval of resected surgical specimens through exploitation of natural body orifices such as the mouth, anus, vagina or urethra.

In this chapter, we described a technique for retrieval of the colonic specimen via a natural orifice or transvaginal for a 78 year old lady who had sigmoid carcinoma and underwent a total laparoscopic high anterior resection, hence avoiding a mini-laparotomy for retrieval of the specimen. We also described various instrumentation and developments in Single Incision Laparoscopic Surgery, NOSE or NOTES, including the latest technique to make this surgery safe. This is concluded with a Health Technology Assessment (HTA) of this emerging technology in health care.

2. Case illustration

2.1 Clinical history

Madam A is a 78 year old lady who complained of per rectal bleeding for 2 months. She had no history of altered bowel habit, loss of appetite or weight and symptoms of bowel obstruction. Examination was unremarkable except for haemorrhoids on proctoscopy. She had a colonoscopy which showed a fungating polypoidal mass at sigmoid colon and biopsy confirmed the lesion to be malignant. Computed Tomography (CT) scan for staging was done and showed no evidence of extra-colonic metastases.

She underwent a total laparoscopic high anterior resection with natural orifice specimen extraction (NOSE) after obtaining an informed consent.

2.2 Operative technique

In the operating theatre, the necessary laparoscopic equipments were readily available. The use of various intracorporeal and extracorporeal stapling devices was also necessary for the operation to be carried out. We also find that the use of Harmonic scalpel ® or ultrasonic dissector to be very useful for tissue dissection during the procedure (Figure 1).

Once patient was placed under general anaesthesia, she was positioned into Lloyd-Davies position. This position allows access to the vagina for specimen retrieval as well as via the anal canal for bowel end to end anastomosis (Figure 2).

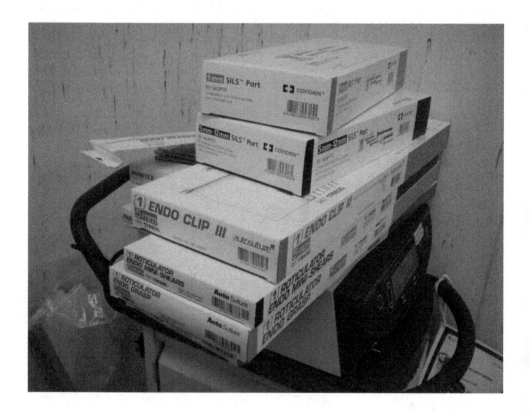

Fig. 1. The various stapling devices, equipments and ultrasonic dissector required for the surgery

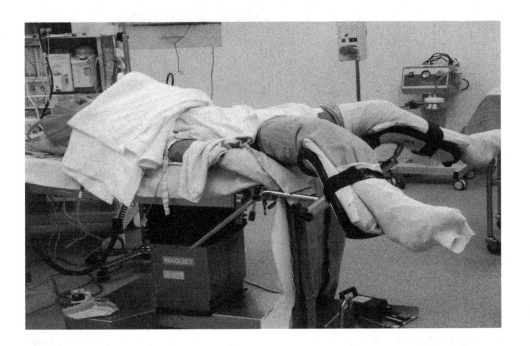

Fig. 2. Positioning of patient for the procedure to be carried out on the operating table.

Intra-operatively, laparoscopic ports were inserted at the appropriate place following pneumoperitoneum. The sigmoid colon was found to be redundant and the tumour was noted to be at the lower sigmoid colon. We began by hitching up the uterus by using a straight needle inserted percutaneously and into the broad ligament of the uterus and retrieving back the needle from the skin where the suture was tied hence lifting the uterus up onto the anterior abdominal wall (Figure 3).

Once there was adequate exposure, we began mobilizing the sigmoid colon from medially to laterally and the left ureter was identified and preserved. The inferior mesenteric vessels were then identified and ligated using vascular staplers. Mesorectal excision was then performed with the tumour further mobilized. The bowel distal to the tumour is then transected using a stapler.

Next, with the assistance from the gynaecologist, the posterior fornix was lifted up using a swab on a sponge forcep that was inserted via the vagina. With the posterior fornix lifted up, a transverse incision is made across the posterior fornix (Figure 4).

The sponge forcep is removed and a laparoscopic hand-port is inserted transvaginally to maintain pneumoperitoneum (Figure 5). The tumour is then delivered transvaginally where it is resected proximally (Figure 6).

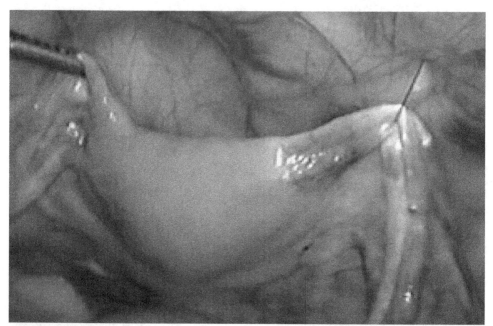

Fig. 3. The uterus hitched to the anterior abdominal wall using sutures passed through the broad ligament

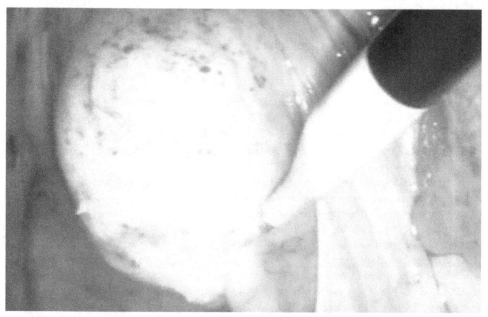

Fig. 4. Incision made across posterior fornix using diathermy following lifting up by the assistant transvaginally

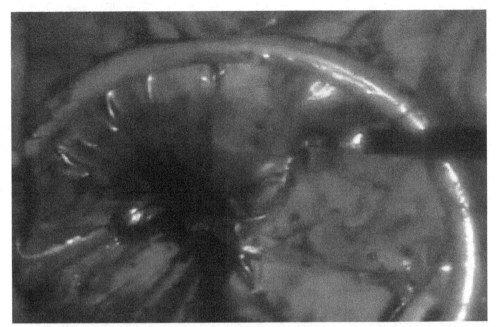

Fig. 5. Hand port inserted via vagina and through the incision made across the posterior fornix. Seen here within the abdomen.

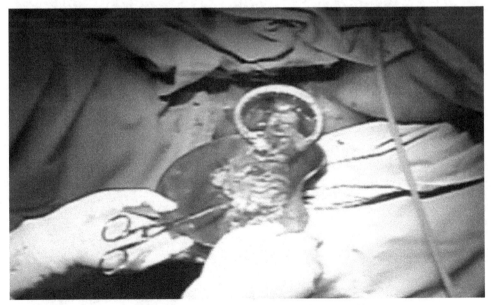

Fig. 6. Tumour extracted out via the vagina and transected proximally to tumour.

The anvil of the circular stapler is then inserted into the proximal colon and closed using purse string suture. The proximal colon is then returned into the abdomen with the anvil. The hand port is removed and the posterior fornix is closed via intracorporeal suturing (Figure 7). Bowel end to end anastomosis was completed by inserting the CDH 29mm circular stapler via anal canal (Figure 8). No leak was encountered intraoperatively when checked post anastomosis.

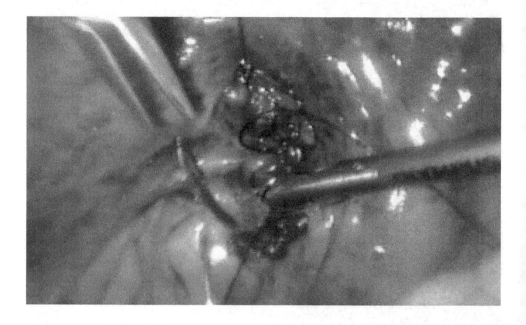

Fig. 7. Posterior fornix is stitched via intracorporeal technique after removal of specimen

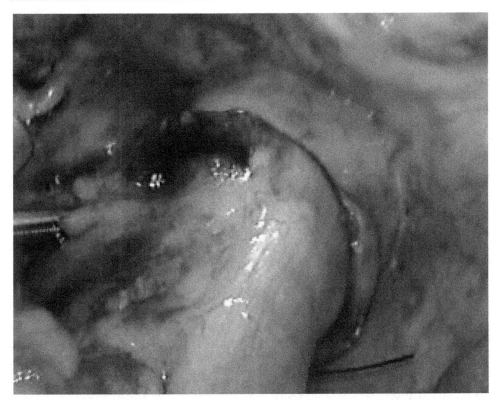

Fig. 8. Bowel end to end anastomosis performed and shown here.

2.3 Clinical progress

Postoperative recovery was uneventful. Pain score was reported to be VAS 0 to 1 throughout her stay. Her post-operative bloods taken did not show any significant changes and blood loss was very minimal. She was put on thrombo-embolic deterrent (TED) stockings, low molecular weight heparin for thromboprophylaxis and was encouraged for incentive spirometry post operatively. We allowed her liquids on the 1st postoperative day and resume normal diet on the 2nd day. There was hardly any post-operative ileus experienced. Her drains were removed at 3rd post-operative day (Figure 9). She began ambulating at day 3 and was discharged on the 5th post-operative day.

On follow up, patient was very happy with the outcome of surgery and was impressed that there was hardly any major scar associated with the operative approach.

2.4 Histopathological result

Histopathological examination showed an 18cm length of colon was removed on gross examination (Figure 10). On microscopic examination, there was no lymphovascular permeation and the tumour only involved the mucosa layer. The margins were clear of tumour. All lymph nodes harvested were negative for malignancy. Proximal and distal donuts were clear of tumour. Pathological staging was noted to be T1, N0, M0 (Stage 1).

The final result showed a moderately differentiated adenocarcinoma.

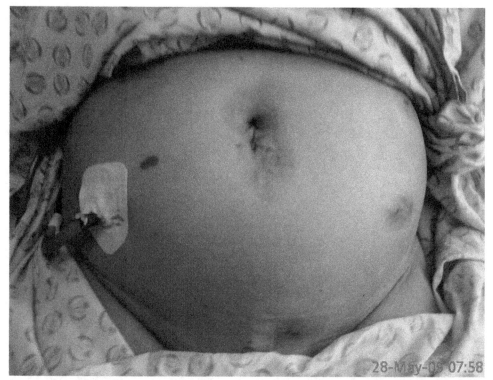

Fig. 9. Wound inspection at post-operative Day 2 showing an almost scarless abdomen

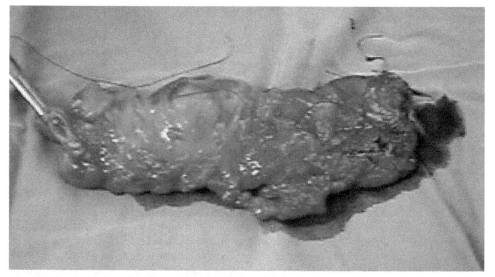

Fig. 10. The entire length of bowel removed along with the tumour.

3. Laparoscopic surgery with Natural Orifice Specimen Extraction (NOSE) in colorectal surgery: The way forward in the scarless surgical approach?

In laparoscopic colorectal resection, it was conventional to retrieve the resected colonic specimen via a mini-laparotomy. This is rather a frustrating situation for most laparoscopic surgeons who took pain to ensure minimal scarring for patients following a long and arduous laparoscopic dissection. Such situation can now be overlooked with the advent of natural orifice surgery, which is gaining popularity and evolving.

It is without doubt that a mini-laparotomy which is required for the retrieval of colonic specimen following resection is associated with a bigger scar hence poor cosmetic appearance, increase in pain outcome, increase risk of wound infection and other pain related complications [1]. This can now be avoided with the technique of retrieving specimens via natural orifices via the transvaginal, transanal or transgastric routes.

In our patient, we have described the retrieval of specimen via the transvaginal route. This is feasible in female patients with colonic cancers. This technique had also been described in other literature. Palanivelu et al. had described the transvaginal route for a series of patients with familial adenosis polyposis (FAP) with early rectal adenocarcinoma who had laparoscopic proctocolectomy with ileoanal pouch anastomosis who had the specimen retrieved transvaginally [2].

Extraction of specimen via the transvaginal route has also been described in other operations besides colorectal surgery such as nephrectomy, cholecystectomy, appendecetomy, spleen and so forth which will be elaborated much later in this chapter [3, 4].

Retrieval of colonic specimen via other natural orifice such as the transgastric or transanal routes had also been described in literature but not without limitations. In this case, the transgastric approach would be limited by the restriction point in the oesophagus, the long travel distance and lack of adequate instruments for extraction as described by Franklin et al [5]. Similarly, the transanal approach also had its limitations such as the risk of fecal contamination, wound infection, injury to the anal sphincters and limitation to the size of the specimen extracted [2, 5]. At this moment, the transanal approach can only be recommended for small benign tumours or early colorectal cancers [6]

One of the reasons for choosing the transvaginal route is the advantage of the elasticity of the vagina, hence allowing specimen of various sizes to be able to retrieve. Literature has shown that transvaginal extraction is most ideal and patients undergoing this technique had good post-operative outcome with clinically no significant impact on orgasm, pregnancy, dyspareunia or sexual function [7].

One of the main concerns regarding retrieval of specimen is port site or retrieval incision metastasis which was reported to be 0.9 to 3.4% by Schaeff et al [8]. However, this fear is allayed as was described in our patient where the use of a handport, which was inserted transvaginally, was used to retrieve the specimen. We also found that the advantage of using the handport also allowed us to minimize infection or contamination, and to maintain pneumoperitoneum throughout the operation.

As can be seen in our patient, the post-recovery was excellent. Pain outcome was good with almost no pain reported. Normal diet was able to resume from the 2nd post-operative day onwards. By the 3rd day, patient was ambulating. On hindsight, patient was actually able to go home on the 3rd post-operative day with the drains removed. We have kept her longer as this was the first case performed in our centre, hence the longer observation period.

The end result of this technique is very satisfactory and patient was highly satisfied with the post-operative outcome.

4. Application of NOSE or NOTES in other surgical disciplines

The sudden rise in interest towards NOSE or NOTES have also seen its application flourished and boomed in various surgical discipline as we moved into the 21st century. Although still in its infancy, it is slowly gaining popularity and clinical acceptance as can be seen in its application in non-colorectal surgery.

4.1 Other general surgical procedures

Although much has been reported regarding the retrieval of colonic specimens be it a right sided colectomy, left sided colectomy or an anterior resection via the more popular natural orifices such as transvaginal or transanal routes, the application of NOSE and NOTES can also be seen in other non-colorectal procedures.

Similar to retrieval of colonic specimen where feasibility is not an option via the transgastric or the transurethral route, the use of NOSE in retrieval of stomach specimen via the transvaginal route had been described by Jeong et al in 2010. This was the first ever description of retrieval of stomach specimen using NOSE method published for early gastric cancer where patients in its series undergone a subtotal gastrectomy [9].

When compared to NOSE in colorectal surgeries, it has been almost 15 years from the first reported extraction of colonic specimen via natural body orifices to its first stomach specimen extraction via NOSE today. Even then, the first NOSE was first described in 1993 by Delvaux et al who removed the gallbladder via the transvaginal route [10]. What have happened along those years?

One can only wonder that such a procedure must have slowly gained acceptance and changed in perception among the clinical community and public acceptance towards NOSE where the procedure can now extend to extraction of other bodily specimens as the people are slowly more inclined towards a scarless surgery.

With regards to NOTES, the use of natural orifices to perform surgery without any bodily incision thus providing patients with a scarless surgery have also been described although it has its limitations. Nevertheless, the future looks promising with the advent of such newer techniques.

At the moment NOTES have been described using an endoscope which is channeled through various bodily orifices and perforating the viscus to perform the intended procedure. Here, examples of peritoneoscopy, appendecectomy, cholecystectomy and so forth had been performed via the transgastric route with retrieval of the specimen. Other routes such as the transcolonic or transvesical or transvaginal route have also been described where once the instruments is in the peritoneal cavity, pneumoperitoneum is created and surgery is performed [11].

In the present, there are still limitations for NOTES when it comes to performing more complex surgery and as for now, most procedures are still performed on animal models. With better technological advancement and improvement in the development of equipments used in NOTES the future indeed looks promising.

4.2 Urology

The use of natural body orifices in Urology began first with the extraction of resected specimen. This was first reported in 1993 by Breda et al following a laparoscopic nephrectomy where the kidney was removed via the transvaginal route [12]. Following this, numerous application of NOSE and NOTES began the flourish in the urological world with popularity began to soar.

The use of transvaginal route for specimen extraction in females was also widely reported by Gill et al who extended the procedure to include radical nephrectomy [13].

Further evidence in the use of other natural orifices slowly took place where the transanal route was used for the extraction of bladder following cystectomy for bladder tumours where a rectosigmoid pouch was created for urinary diversion and the tumour removed via the transanal route [14].

The above described techniques often combined the use of laparoscopic techniques coupled with natural orifice specimen extraction often known as the Hybrid technique. However, pure NOTES where performing surgery via natural orifices without the possibility of any skin incision in Urological procedure began to emerge thus making Urological procedures a complete scarless surgery.

This was first described in animal models but Lima et al in 2006 described the first pure NOTES where peritoneoscopy was done via the transvesical route which allow peritoneal assessment and liver biopsy [15]. The very same author had gone on to describe other surgical procedures using the same transvesical route.

Another urological option towards an almost scarless surgery seems possible with the introduction of Single Incision Laparoscopic Surgery (SILS) making most urological procedure a possibility in using this approach. Of course, we will be touching on about SILS much later in the chapter.

Although it seem like such urological procedures are still a long way from gaining routine acceptance and at times seem experimental, nevertheless the road ahead looks promising. Nevertheless, limitations abound and there is still more work to be done.

4.3 Gynaecological procedures

The emergence of NOSE and NOTES can also be seen in the field of gynaecology. The use of endoscopic procedure via the transvaginal route has established both diagnostic and therapeutic needs in the field of gynaecology. This is better known as culdoscopy among the gynaecology fraternity.

This further transcends towards the use of fertility medicine such as investigation for infertility in both diagnostic and therapeutic means known as Transvaginal Hydrolaparoscopy (THL) [16]. THL is a modification of culdoscopy and was first introduced by Gordts in 1998. It enables the surgeon to assess or evaluate the posterior uterus, the pelvic side walls and adnexae structures. Such procedure acts as a diagnostic tool and can often times be performed under local anaesthesia without subjecting patients to the risk of general anaesthesia.

THL when coupled with chromotubation also allows assessment of infertility and can replace the conventional hysterosalpingography (HSG) which is often used as the first line of diagnostic modality in the assessment of infertility. It is able to show tubal patency as accurately as an HSG.

Besides diagnostic yield, it also allows various operative procedures to be performed such as ovarian drilling, adhesiolysis, treatment of ovarian cyst as well as endometriosis and salpingostomy.

5. Single Incision Laparoscopic Surgery (SILS) the almost scarless surgical approach and the transumbilical route as another natural body orifice?

5.1 SILS experience

Laparoscopic surgery when first introduced in the early 80's brought a revolutionary change to how surgery is performed. Since then, it has evolved from a simple cholecystectomy or appendecectomy to a more complex surgical procedures such as colorectal resection, bariatric surgery, liver and pancreatic resection and so forth.

It is the intention of every laparoscopic surgeon to offer patients with a more feasible form of surgery in the hope of reducing pain, hospital stay and morbidity. Of utmost importance is the reduction or prevention of the conventional surgical scars associated with open surgery. Hence, laparoscopic surgery has evolved from the conventional laparoscopic ports used in certain laparoscopic surgical procedure to usage of much lesser ports for similar procedure.

A fine example is the conventional laparoscopic cholecystectomy with the use of four laparoscopic ports. From thence, literature has been published regarding use of three or even two ports for laparoscopic cholecystectomy with the intention of further reducing the amount of scar as well as tissue damage associated with port insertion [17, 18].

From here, laparoscopic surgery has further evolved when used in combination with NOSE or NOTES to further reduce surgical scars to an almost scarless surgery as was described in this chapter earlier. This is sometimes known as a hybrid procedure. Patients can now be offered this form of surgery as large specimens that cannot be retrieved via the small laparoscopic ports can be retrieved via the natural orifice. This enables us to avoid giving patient a big scar as it made no sense to make a big scar to retrieve specimen that is resected after going through many hours of performing such a complex surgery.

It is only a matter of time when laparoscopic surgery is performed via a single port, hence the introduction of single incision laparoscopic surgery (SILS). This may allow one to do away with some of the combined procedures with NOSE and NOTES as surgery can now be done via one incision with retrieval of specimen from the same incision.

When the single incision or port is inserted via the umbilicus or transumbilical, post-surgical scars is almost invisible when made over the umbilicus. Our experience in our centre has seen SILS being performed for operation such as cholecystectomy (Figure 11), excision of gastric Gastrointestinal stromal tumour (Figure 12), right hemi-colectomy (Figure 13), appendecectomy, SILS anterior resection, SILS spleno-distal pancreatectomy and inguinal hernia repair where the port is inserted via theumbilicus. Post operatively, these scars were almost invisible or in other words scarless! Patients who have undergone these procedures were very satisfied with the outcome of this surgery and were happy that almost no scars were noticeable. Recovery is often uneventful and patients have experienced lower amount of pain.

In some literature, the umbilical route has also been described as a natural orifice as it is considered once as a natural orifice during embryological development. Hence, the term natural orifice transumbilical surgery (NOTUS) has been coined [19].

Not to rest on its laurels, SILS has also seen itself being evolved into more complex surgery such as colorectal resections or even bariartric surgery. The uses of SILS have also been described in various urological and gynaecological procedures as well with favourable outcomes.

Chambers et al have described the use of SILS in various colorectal resections ranging from appendecectomy to hemicolectomies and anterior resection and proved that it was a safe and feasible surgery to perform in the hands of experience surgeons [20]. With regards to bariartric surgery, Reavis et al have described how sleeve gastrectomy was performed in obesity surgery via a single incision for laparoscopic ports placement and retrieval of the stomach specimen via the same incision [21].

The various literatures published to date regarding SILS augurs well for this surgical technology to further develop and as an offering to patients seeking a scarless surgery in the near future.

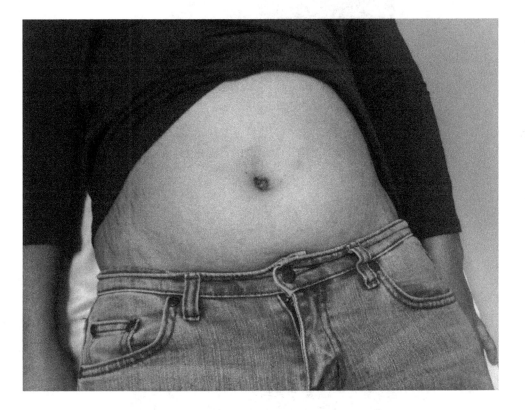

Fig. 11. Almost scarless wound at the umbilicus after SILS cholecystectomy

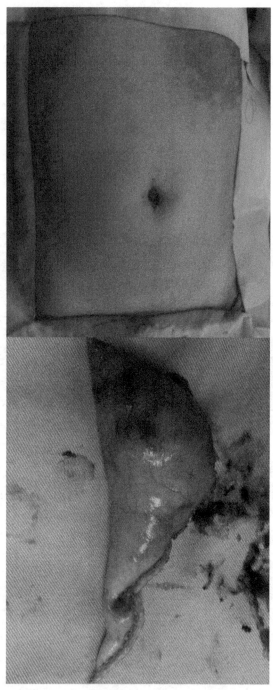

Fig. 12. Almost scarless wound at the umbilicus after SILS wedge excision of gastric GIST

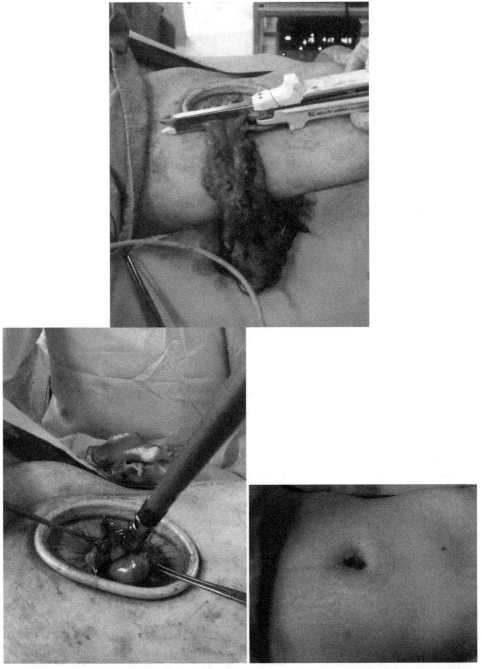

Fig. 13. An almost scarless wound at the umbilicus after a SILS right hemi-colectomy with extracorporeal anastomosis as demonstrated above.

5.2 The challenge ahead for SILS

Like any new surgical technology, SILS is not without its limitations. Among the many challenges faced by surgeons taking up SILS is the associated long learning curve. It is believed that one may overcome this limitation as more experience is gained from performing SILS on a regular basis.

More young surgeons should also be encouraged to take up this procedure as the longer exposure to SILS will in turn be gained as an experience over a period of time.

Next would be the instrumentation associated with SILS. The smaller degree of instrument triangulation often hampers or discourages one from taking up SILS. In our experience, this is one major drawback to SILS as oftentimes, surgeons finds it difficult to perform SILS with the conventional and existing available instruments. It is not without doubt that smaller degrees of instrument triangulation often occurs compared to the conventional laparoscopic procedures when a single port is used. However, this may be overcome with better laparoscopic ports, platforms and devices which may allow flexibility and angulation to facilitate the use of SILS. This has actually encouraged industry players to inject funds into research and development for better instruments and equipment related to SILS as can be seen in today's modern day of surgical practice.

Is the future looking bright for SILS? We believe so, albeit a learning curve is associated with it and future development of newer laparoscopic instruments may further enhance and ease the use of this new surgical technology as more and more patients demand for a scarless approach to surgery in the near future.

6. Conclusion

The transvaginal route is most ideal for the retrieval of colonic specimens in laparoscopic colorectal surgery due to the advantage of its anatomical and physiological properties. Our experience with this technique showed that it is feasible for selected patients. It is also a safe procedure with low morbidity. Pain outcome is good and patient satisfaction is excellent.

The use of NOSE can also been seen in its application in other surgical disciplines allowing specimen extraction using various routes described.

Other techniques such as NOTES and SILS have also gained popularity and acceptance in this fast moving day and age of surgical technologies. These techniques described above often times complement each other or may be accomplished on its own in the case of SILS.

In conclusion, the advancement and evolution in surgical techniques this present day and for the future gives patients the satisfaction of an almost a scarless surgery.

7. References

[1] Cheung, H.Y., et al., *Endo-laparoscopic colectomy without mini-laparotomy for left sided colonic tumors.* World J Surg, 2009. 33(6): p. 1287-1291.

[2] Palanivelu, C., et al., *An innovative technique for colorectal specimen retrieval: A new era for Natural Orifice Specimen Extraction (NOSE)*. Diseases of the Colon and Rectum, 2008. 51: p. 1120-1124.

[3] Gill, I.S., et al., *Vaginal extraction of the intact specimen following laparoscopic radical nephrectomy*. J Urol, 2002. 167: p. 238-241.

[4] Vereczkei, A., et al., *Transvaginal extraction of the laparoscopically removed spleen*. Surg Endosc, 2003. 17: p. 157.

[5] Franklin, M.E., et al., *Transvaginal extraction of the specimen after total laparoscopic right hemicolectomy with intracorporeal anastomosis*. Surg Laparosc Endosc Percutan Tech, 2008. 18(3): p. 294-298.

[6] Ooi, B.S., et al., *Laparoscopic high anterior resection with natural orifice specimen extraction (NOSE) for early rectal cancer*. Tech Coloproctol 2009. 13: p. 61-64.

[7] Roovers, J.P., et al., *A randomized comparison of post operative pain, quality of life, and physical performance during the first six weeks after abdominal or vaginal surgery correction of the uteri*. Neurourol Urodyn, 2005. 24: p. 334–340.

[8] Schaeff, B., V. Paolucci, and J. Thomopoulos, *Port site recurrences after laparoscopic surgery. A review*. Dig Surg 1998. 15: p. 124–134.

[9] Jeong, S.H., et al., *Trans-vaginal specimen extraction following totally laparoscopic subtotal gastrectomy in early gastric cancer*. Gastric Cancer, 2011. 14(1): p. 91-6.

[10] Delvaux, G., et al., *Transvaginal removal of gallbladders with large stones after laparoscopic cholecystectomy*. Surg Laparosc Endosc, 1993. 3(4): p. 307-9.

[11] Pearl, J.P. and J.L. Ponsky, *Natural orifice translumenal endoscopic surgery: a critical review*. J Gastrointest Surg, 2008. 12(7): p. 1293-300.

[12] Breda, G., et al., *Laparoscopic nephrectomy with vaginal delivery of the intact kidney*. Eur Urol, 1993. 24(1): p. 116-7.

[13] Gill, I.S., et al., *Vaginal extraction of the intact specimen following laparoscopic radical nephrectomy*. J Urol, 2002. 167(1): p. 238-41.

[14] DeGer, S., et al., *Laparoscopic radical cystectomy with continent urinary diversion (rectosigmoid pouch) performed completely intracorporeally: an intermediate functional and oncologic analysis*. Urology, 2004. 64(5): p. 935-9.

[15] Lima, E., et al., *Transvesical endoscopic peritoneoscopy: a novel 5 mm port for intra-abdominal scarless surgery*. J Urol, 2006. 176(2): p. 802-5.

[16] Escobar, P.F., et al., *Laparoendoscopic single-site and natural orifice surgery in gynecology*. Fertil Steril, 2010. 94(7): p. 2497-502.

[17] Kagaya, T., *Laparoscopic cholecystectomy via two ports, using the "Twin-Port" system*. J Hepatobiliary Pancreat Surg, 2001. 8(1): p. 76-80.

[18] Leggett, P.L., et al., *Three-port microlaparoscopic cholecystectomy in 159 patients*. Surg Endosc, 2001. 15(3): p. 293-6.

[19] Nguyen, N.T., et al., *Laparoscopic transumbilical cholecystectomy without visible abdominal scars*. J Gastrointest Surg, 2009. 13(6): p. 1125-8.

[20] Chambers, W.M., et al., *Single-incision laparoscopic surgery (SILS) in complex colorectal surgery: a technique offering potential and not just cosmesis*. Colorectal Dis, 2011. 13(4): p. 393-8.

[21] Reavis, K.M., et al., *Single-laparoscopic incision transabdominal surgery sleeve gastrectomy.* Obes Surg, 2008. 18(11): p. 1492-4.

10

Microbial Contamination of Suction Tubes Attached to Suction Instrument and Its Preventive Methods

Katsuhiro Yorioka[1] and Shigeharu Oie[2]
*[1]Department of Pharmacy, Shunan Municipal Shinnanyo
Citizen Hospital, 2-3-15 Miyanomae, Shunan
[2]Department of Pharmacy, Yamaguchi University
Hospital; 1-1-1 Minamikogushi, Ube
Japan*

1. Introduction

We investigated the microbial contamination of suction tubes attached to wall-type suction instrument. Microbial contamination of suction tubes used for endoscopy or sputum suction in wards was examined before and after their disinfection. In addition, disinfection and washing methods for suction tubes were evaluated. Suction tubes (N=33) before disinfection were contaminated with 10^2-10^8 colony-forming units (cfu) / tube. The main contaminants were *Pseudomonas aeruginosa*, *Acinetobacter baumannii*, and *Stenotrophomonas maltophilia*. The suction tubes were disinfected with sodium hypochlorite (N=11) or hot water (N=11), or using an automatic tube cleaner (N=11). After 2-hour immersion in 0.1% (1,000 ppm) sodium hypochlorite, 10^3-10^7cfu/tube of bacteria were detected in all 11 tubes examined. After washing in hot running water (65°C), 10^3-10^7cfu / tube were detected in 3 of 11 examined tubes. The bacteria detected in the suction tubes after disinfection with sodium hypochlorite or hot water were *P. aeruginosa*, *A.baumannii*, and *S.maltophilia*. On the other hand, after washing with warm water (40°C) using the automatic tube cleaner, the contamination were < 20 cfu / tube (lower detection limit: 20 cfu / tube) in all 11 tubes examined. These results suggest the usefulness of washing using the automatic tube cleaners.

2. Background

In hospitals in Japan, the suction of body fluid such as sputum or blood is performed daily using wall-type suction instrument in wards and outpatient clinics such as endoscopy rooms (**Fig.1-a,2-b**). Wall-mounted suction instrument are used being connected to a suction tube. Suction instruments are used for procedures such as sputum suction, endoscopy using a suction tube connected to a gastrofiberscope, and bronchoalveolar lavage (BAL) using a suction tube connected to a bronchofiberscope. In sputum suction and suction in gastrofiberscopy, sucked body fluid (such as sputum and saliva) flows from the patient's

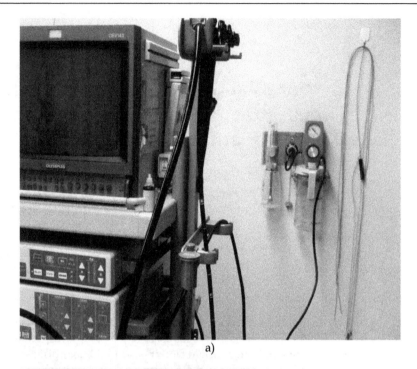

a)

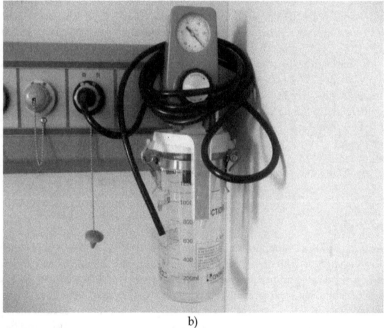

b)

Fig. 1.

side toward the suction tube (suction instruments). However, in BAL, regurgitation from the suction tube side toward the bronchofiberscope or bronchoalveolar lavage fluid (BALF) sometimes occurs (1). Indeed, we experienced regurgitation from the suction tube side toward the BALF side several times during BAL. BAL using suction tubes that are contaminated or have not been disinfected runs the risk of the contamination of patients and BALF, which may induce nosocomial infection (2, 3). When suction tubes are washed or disinfected in sink such as the ward or outpatient clinic, water drops containing patients' body fluid and microorganism's splash on health care workers, which runs the risk of exposure and infection (4-6). The use of disposable (single-use) suction tubes or washing/disinfection of suction tubes in each patient is necessary. However, at present, there are no guidelines (or recommendation) regarding the washing/disinfection methods for suction tubes as non-critical instruments. In addition, there are no clinical data on the relationship between the microbial contamination of suction tubes and their disinfection methods. Therefore, we evaluated microbial contamination of suction tubes and methods for their disinfection.

3. Methods

We investigated the microbial contamination of suction tubes that are used, being connected to wall-type suction instruments (Central Uni Co., Tokyo, Japan), and evaluated their disinfection/washing methods. Microbial contamination in a total of 33 suction tubes used for endoscopy or sputum suction in wards was compared before and after disinfection/washing. Tubes were disinfected with sodium hypochlorite (N=11) or hot water (N=11), or washed using an automatic tube cleaner (N=11). Per one patient, we used one suction tube. The suction tube is 3m in length, 4mm in internal diameter and made of high-purity latex (Deluxe type latex tubing: Central Uni Co., Tokyo, Japan). The washing methods using sodium hypochlorite, hot water, or an automatic tube cleaner are as follows.

Disinfection with sodium hypochlorite solution: Suction tubes after use were washed under running water, immersed in 0.1% (1,000 ppm) sodium hypochlorite for 2 hours (**Fig.2-a**), and dried naturally in the ward or endoscopy room.

Disinfection with hot water: Suction tubes were washed under running water and immersed in an enzyme detergent (Biotect®55, Sakura Seiki Co.,Tokyo, Japan) at 40°C for 30 minutes. Subsequently, hot water (65°C) was run into the suction tubes for 5 minutes (**Fig.2-b**). In addition, the tubes were flushed with 20 mL of 80% (v/v) ethanol for disinfection (Yoshida Pharmaceutical Co., Tokyo, Japan) using a syringe, and dried naturally in the ward.

Washing using an automatic tube cleaner: Suction tubes were washed using an automatic tube cleaner in the central supply room, flushed with 20 mL of 80% (v/v) ethanol for disinfection, and dried using an automatic drier at 70°C for 2 hours. This automatic tube cleaner automatically performs the cleaning process consisting of washing with an enzyme detergent, washing without a detergent, rinsing, and drying (**Fig.2-c**: Automatic tube cleaner MU-72 K: Sharp System Product Co.,Tokyo, Japan). Warm water at 40°C, with which the optimal effects of the enzyme detergent can be expected, was used for the automatic tube cleaner.

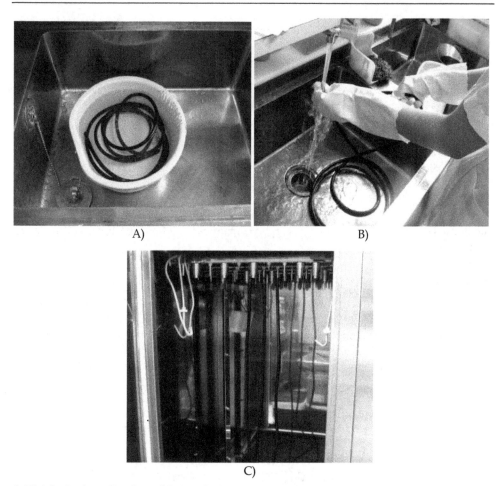

A: Disinfection by sodium hypochlorite solution
Suction tubes after use were washed under running tap water, immersed in 0.1% (1,000 ppm) sodium hypochlorite for 2 hours.
B: Disinfection with hot water
Suction tubes were washed under running tap water and immersed in an enzyme detergent at 40°C for 30 minutes. Subsequently, hot water (65°C) was run into the suction tubes for 5 minutes.
C: Washing with an automatic tube cleaner
This automatic tube cleaner automatically performs the cleaning process consisting of   washing with an enzyme detergent, washing without a detergent, rinsing, and drying.

Fig. 2. Immersion in sodium hypochlorite (a), washing under running hot water (b) and washing with an automatic tube cleaner (c)

4. Results

Table 1 shows the results of microbial contamination in suction tubes before disinfection with immersion in sodium hypochlorite solution, washing with hot water, and washing with an automatic tube cleaner. Suction tubes before disinfection with sodium hypochlorite solution or hot water were contaminated with 10^3-10^8 cfu/tube, and the main contaminants were *Pseudomonas aeruginosa, Acinetobacter baumannii,* and *Stenotrophomonas maltophilia*. Table 2 shows the results of microbial contamination in suction tubes after disinfection by immersion in sodium hypochlorite solution, those after washing by hot running water, and those after washing with warm water using an automatic tube cleaner. Bacteria were detected in all 11 examined tubes after 2-hour immersion in 0.1% (1,000 ppm) sodium hypochlorite solution and 3 of 11 after washing in hot running water. The contaminant after disinfection was 10^3-10^8 cfu/tube, and the contaminants detected in the suction tubes were glucose non-fermentative gram-negative rods such as *P. aeruginosa, A. baumannii, Sphingomonas paucimobilis,* and *Stenotrophomonas maltophilia*. The contaminant was < 20 cfu/tube (lower detection limit, 20 cfu/tube) in all 11 examined tubes after washing using the automatic tube cleaner.

After disinfection by immersion in sodium hypochlorite solution or washing in hot running water, 14 (63.6%) of the 22 tubes examined were contaminated with 10^3-10^7 cfu/tube. The main contaminants were glucose non-fermentative gram-negative rods such as *Pseudomonas aeruginosa, Acinetobacter baumannii,* and *Stenotrophomonas maltophilia*.

5. Discussion

This inadequate disinfection may be because the inside of the tubes was not immersed in sodium hypochlorite solution due to the thin long tube structure (≥ 3 m), and organic matter and microorganisms in the tubes could not be removed or diluted, and remained. Indeed, in a suction tube after disinfection by immersion in sodium hypochlorite solution, a mass of body fluid was discovered (**Fig.3**). On the other hand, all 11 automatic tube cleaners examined were contaminated with < 20 cfu/tube, showing accurate disinfection effects. Automatic cleaners can reduce microorganisms and organic matter inside suction tubes by a mean of 4 log (99.9%) **(7)**. The use of automatic cleaners is a useful disinfection method that has marked disinfection effects without causing side effects due to residual toxicity, as are observed with disinfectants **(8)**.

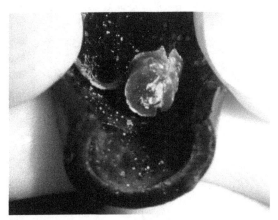

Fig. 3. A mass of body fluid discovered in the suction tube after disinfection with sodium hypochlorite solution.

Table 1. Microbial contamination inside suction tubes before disinfection with sodium hypochlorite solution, disinfection with hot water, or washing using automatic tube cleaner

before disinfection with sodium hypochlorite

Sample No.	Colony (CFU/tube)	Contaminants
1	$2.4×10^3$	Escherichia coli
2	$2.7×10^7$	Klebsiella oxytoca
	$2.2×10^4$	Acinetobacter baumannii
	$2.0×10^7$	Stenotrophomonas maltophilia
3	$8.0×10^4$	Pseudomonas aeruginosa
	$3.5×10^6$	Acinetobacter baumannii
	$8.4×10^5$	Sphingobacterium multivorum
4	$2.8×10^5$	Acinetobacter baumannii
	$7.2×10^5$	Sphingobacterium multivorum
	$5.5×10^5$	Stenotrophomonas maltophilia
5	$3.5×10^6$	Acinetobacter baumannii
	$1.4×10^6$	Sphingobacterium multivorum
6	$1.3×10^8$	Acinetobacter baumannii
	$1.0×10^7$	Pseudomonas pertucinogena
	$3.2×10^6$	Escherichia coli
7	$4.2×10^2$	Pseudomonas pertucinogena
	$1.5×10^3$	Acinetobacter baumannii
	$6.0×10^4$	Escherichia coli
8	$2.3×10^8$	Acinetobacter baumannii
9	$1.2×10^7$	Pseudomonas pertucinogena
	$6.5×10^8$	Stenotrophomonas maltophilia
	$4.5×10^7$	Chryseobacterium meningosepticum
10	$2.0×10^5$	Pseudomonas aeruginosa
	$3.0×10^6$	Pseudomonas oryzihabitans
11	$6.4×10^4$	Stenotrophomonas maltophilia
	$2.6×10^5$	Chryseobacterium meningosepticum

before disinfection with hot water

Sample No.	Colony (CFU/tube)	Contaminants
1	$5.5×10^5$	Acinetobacter baumannii
2	$3.6×10^4$	Pseudomonas aeruginosa
	$3.0×10^3$	Stenotrophomonas maltophilia
3	$4.4×10^7$	Pseudomonas aeruginosa
	$2.5×10^6$	Acinetobacter baumannii
4	$3.4×10^5$	Acinetobacter lwoffii
	$3.0×10^5$	Chryseobacterium meningosepticum
5	$4.5×10^6$	Acinetobacter baumannii
	$5.0×10^3$	Pseudomonas aeruginosa
6	$3.0×10^4$	Acinetobacter lwoffii
7	$6.0×10^5$	Stenotrophomonas maltophilia
	$4.2×10^6$	Pseudomonas aeruginosa
	$2.7×10^3$	Acinetobacter baumannii
8	$7.0×10^6$	Pseudomonas aeruginosa
	$8.0×10^7$	Sphingomonas paucimobilis
	$3.5×10^6$	Acinetobacter lwoffii
9	$5.0×10^4$	Stenotrophomonas maltophilia
10	$2.1×10^7$	Chryseobacterium meningosepticum
11	$4.8×10^6$	Pseudomonas aeruginosa
	$5.3×10^5$	Pseudomonas aeruginosa
	$2.0×10^7$	Acinetobacter calcoaceticus

before washing with automatic tube cleaner

Sample No.	Colony (CFU/tube)	Contaminants
1	$3.0×10^6$	Acinetobacter baumannii
2	$3.0×10^5$	Stenotrophomonas maltophilia
	$4.4×10^8$	Pseudomonas aeruginosa
3	$2.6×10^7$	Acinetobacter lwoffii
4	$2.0×10^4$	Acinetobacter baumannii
	$2.4×10^6$	Pseudomonas aeruginosa
	$5.8×10^5$	Sphingobacterium multivorum
5	$3.0×10^8$	Acinetobacter baumannii
	$5.0×10^3$	Pseudomonas aeruginosa
6	$1.0×10^5$	Sphingomonas paucimobilis
	$1.0×10^7$	Stenotrophomonas maltophilia
7	$4.8×10^5$	Pseudomonas aeruginosa
	$5.0×10^4$	Acinetobacter haemolyticus
	$6.0×10^2$	Acinetobacter baumannii
8	$2.3×10^7$	Pseudomonas aeruginosa
	$8.0×10^7$	Sphingomonas paucimobilis
9	$5.8×10^5$	Stenotrophomonas maltophilia
	$6.6×10^6$	Acinetobacter baumannii
10	$7.8×10^4$	Pseudomonas aeruginosa
	$2.8×10^5$	Stenotrophomonas maltophilia
	$3.6×10^6$	Acinetobacter lwoffii
	$4.4×10^7$	Pseudomonas aeruginosa
11	$6.4×10^4$	Stenotrophomonas maltophilia
	$3.8×10^6$	Acinetobacter baumannii

Table 2. Microbial contamination inside suction tubes after disinfection with sodium hypochlorite solution, disinfection with hot water, or washing using automatic tube cleaner

after disinfection with sodium hypochlorite

Sample No.	Colony (CFU/tube)	Contaminants
1	4.2×10^5	Pseudomonas aeruginosa
2	2.0×10^4	Pseudomonas aeruginosa
	2.0×10^4	Acinetobacter baumannii
	7.4×10^5	Stenotrophomonas maltophilia
	1.2×10^6	Sphingomonas paucimobilis
3	1.2×10^4	Pseudomonas aeruginosa
	3.6×10^4	Acinetobacter baumannii
	3.4×10^5	Sphingobacterium multivorum
	7.2×10^5	Sphingomonas paucimobilis
4	6.0×10^5	Acinetobacter baumannii
	4.0×10^5	Pseudomonas aeruginosa
	1.1×10^7	Sphingobacterium multivorum
5	1.2×10^4	Acinetobacter baumannii
	1.6×10^3	Pseudomonas aeruginosa
	6.6×10^4	Sphingobacterium multivorum
6	8.4×10^5	Pseudomonas aeruginosa
	2.8×10^6	Stenotrophomonas maltophilia
7	8.0×10^4	Pseudomonas aeruginosa
	6.4×10^5	Sphingomonas paucimobilis
	4.8×10^5	Stenotrophomonas maltophilia
8	8.0×10^3	Pseudomonas aeruginosa
	1.6×10^4	Acinetobacter baumannii
	1.5×10^5	Stenotrophomonas maltophilia
	5.1×10^5	Sphingomonas paucimobilis
9	3.2×10^6	Stenotrophomonas maltophilia
	6.8×10^6	Chryseobacterium meningosepticum
10	4.0×10^3	Pseudomonas oryzihabitans
	2.0×10^4	Empedobacter brevis
11	4.8×10^6	Stenotrophomonas maltophilia
	4.0×10^6	Chryseobacterium meningosepticum

after disinfection with hot water

Sample No.	Colony (CFU/tube)*	Contaminants
1	< 20	—
2	< 20	—
3	7.2×10^3	Acinetobacter baumannii
4	< 20	—
5	1.6×10^7	Pseudomonas aeruginosa
	4.4×10^6	Stenotrophomonas maltophilia
6	< 20	—
7	< 20	—
8	1.0×10^6	Pseudomonas aeruginosa
	3.2×10^5	Acinetobacter lwoffii
9	< 20	—
10	< 20	—
11	< 20	—

after washing with automatic tube cleaner

Sample No.	Colony (CFU/tube)*	Contaminants
1	< 20	—
2	< 20	—
3	< 20	—
4	< 20	—
5	< 20	—
6	< 20	—
7	< 20	—
8	< 20	—
9	< 20	—
10	< 20	—
11	< 20	—

*Lower detection limit: 20 cfu/tube

The present status survey in the 18 institutions revealed 3 institutions (16%) using disposable tubes and 2 (11%) (including our hospital) where the disinfection of tubes is performed (by immersion in sodium hypochlorite at the ward/outpatient clinic in both institutions). When moist/respiratory tract medical instruments such as suction tube are disinfected at the ward or outpatient clinic, medial workers or sinks are contaminated with water droplets from suction tubes, which may cause occupational infection (9-11). On the other hand, washing with automatic tube cleaners is certain decontamination/washing effects than the disinfection method performed at the ward or outpatient clinic, and is also desirable in terms of the prevention of occupational contamination of medical workers performing washing/disinfection (12-13). Therefore, it is necessary to recommend the use of disposable suction tubes or washing disinfection using automatic tube cleaners by medical staff members of the central supply room.

6. References

[1] The European society of pneumology task group on BAL. (1990): Eur. Respir. J., 3, 937-974.

[2] Wishart, M.M., Riley, T.V. (1967): Infection with *Pseudomonas maltophilia* hospital outbreak due to contaminated disinfectant. Med. J. Aust., 2, 710−712.

[3] Pokrywka, M., Viazanko, K., Medvick, J. et al. (1993): A *Flavobacterium meningosepticum* outbreak among intensive care paitients. Am. J. Infect. Control., 21, 139−145.

[4] Ferroni, A., Nguyen, L., Pron, B., Quesne, G., Brussent, M.C., Berche, P. (1998): Oubreak of nosocomial urinary tract infection due to *Pseudomonas aeruginosa* in a pediatric sur-gical unit associated with tap-water contamination. J. Hosp. Infect., 39, 301-307.

[5] Widmer, A.F., Wenzel, R.P., Trilla, A., Bale, M.J., Jones, R.N., Doebbeling, B.N. (1993): Outbreaks of *Pseudomonas aeruginosa* infections in a surgical intensive care unit: probable transmission via hands of a health care worker. Clin. Infect. Dis., 16, 372-376.

[6] Miller, D.M., Youkhana, I., Karunaratne, W.U., Pearce, A. (2001): Presence of protein deposits on 'cleaned' re-usable anaesthetic equipment. Anaesthesai., 56, 1069−1072.

[7] Rutala, W.A. (1996): APIC guideline for selection and use of disinfectants. Am. J. Infect. Control, 24, 313−342.

[8] Block, C., Baron, O., Bogokowski, B., et al. (1990): An in-use evaluation of decontamination of polypropylene versus steel bedpans. J. Hosp. Infect., 16, 331-338.

[9] Tordoff, S.G., Scott, S. (2002): Blood contamination of the laryngeal mask airways and laryngoscopes-what do we tell our patients? Anaesthesai., 57, 505−506.

[10] (Coetzee, G.J. (2003): Eliminating protein from reusable laryngeal mask airways. A study comparing routinely cleaned masks with three alternative cleaning methods. Anaesthesai., 58, 346−353.

[11] Bodey, G.P., Bolivar, R., Fainstein, V., Jadeja, L.(1983): Infection caused by *Pseudomonas aeruginosa*. Rev. Infect. Dis., 5, 279−313.

[12] Quinn, J.P. (1998): Clinical problems posed by multiresistant nonfermenting gram − negative pathogens. Clin. Infect. Dis., 27, 117−124.

[13] Bergogne-Berezin, E., Towner, K.J. (1996): *Acinetobacter* spp. as nosocomial pathogens: microbiological, clinical, and epidermiological features.Clin. Microbiol. Rev., 148−165.

Permissions

The contributors of this book come from diverse backgrounds, making this book a truly international effort. This book will bring forth new frontiers with its revolutionizing research information and detailed analysis of the nascent developments around the world.

We would like to thank Cornel Iancu, MD, PhD, for lending his expertise to make the book truly unique. He has played a crucial role in the development of this book. Without his invaluable contribution this book wouldn't have been possible. He has made vital efforts to compile up to date information on the varied aspects of this subject to make this book a valuable addition to the collection of many professionals and students.

This book was conceptualized with the vision of imparting up-to-date information and advanced data in this field. To ensure the same, a matchless editorial board was set up. Every individual on the board went through rigorous rounds of assessment to prove their worth. After which they invested a large part of their time researching and compiling the most relevant data for our readers. Conferences and sessions were held from time to time between the editorial board and the contributing authors to present the data in the most comprehensible form. The editorial team has worked tirelessly to provide valuable and valid information to help people across the globe.

Every chapter published in this book has been scrutinized by our experts. Their significance has been extensively debated. The topics covered herein carry significant findings which will fuel the growth of the discipline. They may even be implemented as practical applications or may be referred to as a beginning point for another development. Chapters in this book were first published by InTech; hereby published with permission under the Creative Commons Attribution License or equivalent.

The editorial board has been involved in producing this book since its inception. They have spent rigorous hours researching and exploring the diverse topics which have resulted in the successful publishing of this book. They have passed on their knowledge of decades through this book. To expedite this challenging task, the publisher supported the team at every step. A small team of assistant editors was also appointed to further simplify the editing procedure and attain best results for the readers.

Our editorial team has been hand-picked from every corner of the world. Their multi-ethnicity adds dynamic inputs to the discussions which result in innovative outcomes. These outcomes are then further discussed with the researchers and contributors who give their valuable feedback and opinion regarding the same. The feedback is then collaborated with the researches and they are edited in a comprehensive manner to aid the understanding of the subject.

Apart from the editorial board, the designing team has also invested a significant amount of their time in understanding the subject and creating the most relevant covers. They scrutinized every image to scout for the most suitable representation of the subject and create an appropriate cover for the book.

The publishing team has been involved in this book since its early stages. They were actively engaged in every process, be it collecting the data, connecting with the contributors or procuring relevant information. The team has been an ardent support to the editorial, designing and production team. Their endless efforts to recruit the best for this project, has resulted in the accomplishment of this book. They are a veteran in the field of academics and their pool of knowledge is as vast as their experience in printing. Their expertise and guidance has proved useful at every step. Their uncompromising quality standards have made this book an exceptional effort. Their encouragement from time to time has been an inspiration for everyone.

The publisher and the editorial board hope that this book will prove to be a valuable piece of knowledge for researchers, students, practitioners and scholars across the globe.

List of Contributors

Filippo Tosato, Salvatore Marano, Stefano Mattacchione, Barbara Luongo, Giulia Paltrinieri and Valentina Mingarelli
Referral Center for the Surgical Treatment of Gastroesophageal Reflux Diseases, "Sapienza" University of Rome, Italy

Leoluca Vasapollo
Sandro Pertini Hospital, Rome, Italy

Giuseppe P. Ferulano
Department of Systemic Pathology General and Miniinvasive Surgical Unit, University of Naples "Federico II", Italy

Saverio Dilillo, Michele D'Ambra, Ruggero Lionetti, Piero Di Silverio, Stefano Capasso, Domenico Pelaggi and Michele Rutigliano
Department of Systemic Pathology General and Miniinvasive Surgical Unit (Prof. G.P.Ferulano) University of Naples "Federico II", Italy

Karim M. Eltawil
Dalhousie University, Department of Surgery, Queen Elizabeth II Health Sciences Centre, Rm 6-302 Victoria Building, Halifax, Nova Scotia, Canada

Michele Molinari
Associate Professor of Surgery, Rm 6-302 Victoria Building, Halifax, Nova Scotia, Canada

Coco Claudio, Rizzo Gianluca, Verbo Alessandro, Mattana Claudio, Pafundi Donato Paolo and Manno Alberto
Catholic University of the Sacred Heart, Department of Surgical Sciences, Rome, Italy

Rastislav Hejj, Marie McNulty and John G. Calleary
Department of Urology, North Manchester General Hospital, Pennine Acute Hospitals, NHS Trust Crumpsall, Manchester M8 5RB, United Kingdom

Marco Berlucchi and Barbara Pedruzzi
Department of Pediatric Otorhinolaryngology, Spedali Civili, Brescia, Italy

Michele Sessa and Piero Nicolai
Department of Otolaryngology, University of Brescia, Brescia, Italy

Kris R. Jatana
Nationwide Children's Hospital and The Ohio State University Columbus, Ohio, USA

Jeffrey C. Rastatter
Children's Memorial Hospital and Northwestern University Chicago, Illinois, USA

Ivana Pajić-Penavić
Department of ENT, Head and Neck Surgery, General Hospital "Dr Josip Benčević", Slavonski Brod, Croatia

Peng Soon Koh and Kin Fah Chin
Department of Surgery, Faculty of Medicine, University of Malaya, Kuala Lumpur, Malaysia

Katsuhiro Yorioka
Department of Pharmacy, Shunan Municipal Shinnanyo Citizen Hospital, 2-3-15 Miyanomae, Shunan

Shigeharu Oie
Department of Pharmacy, Yamaguchi University Hospital; 1-1-1 Minamikogushi, Ube, Japan

Printed in the USA
CPSIA information can be obtained
at www.ICGtesting.com
JSHW011412221024
72173JS00003B/516